A Pharm

An authentic tale of true love, family, addiction, and the practice of pharmacy.

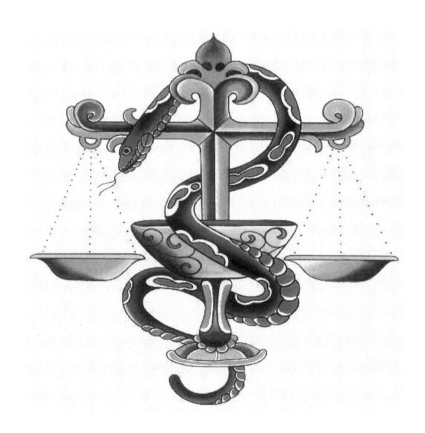

Steve Leuck, Pharm.D.

The title page picture is an original piece of art, designed by a tattoo artist in Santa Cruz, California, specifically to celebrate my 15th year of sobriety. Prominently placed on my left shoulder, I am nearing my third decade, one-day-at-a-time.

The Bowl of Hygeia is a recognized symbol of pharmacy that originated in Greek mythology. Hygeia was the daughter and assistant of Aesculapius, the god of Medicine and Healing. The classic symbol of Hygeia is a bowl containing medicinal potion with the Serpent of Wisdom guarding it. The Pharmacy Scales are a more recent symbol of pharmacy and healing.

The Bowl of Hygeia, the Serpent of Wisdom and the Pharmacy Scales combine to provide a symbol that, in my opinion, depicts a balanced and unwavering understanding of healing through medication.

Dedication

Importantly, more than anything else, this book is a dedication to the love of my life, Susie. From each page through every chapter, Susie is with me. Her devotion to family, quintessential sensitivity, passion for lifelong learning and unwavering love of her children and husband make me, daily, strive to be a better human. Susie is my lighthouse, without her, I absolutely would not be where I am today.

Steve

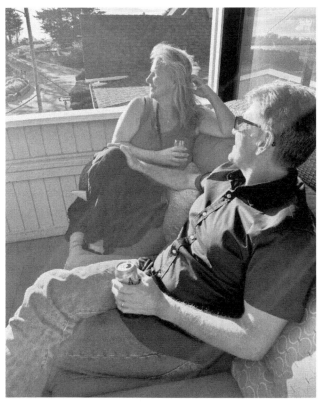

Photo courtesy of Bronwyn Fargo.

Contents

Forward

Innumerable times, over the past many years, I have meditated about beginning to draft my story. Attempting to reconstruct the stories of nearly four decades feels like an incredibly long walk around a large barn; however, for reasons which I will disclose in these pages, now is the time for me to begin.

This is my attempt at navigating, with words, my feelings and life changing moments since I graduated high school in 1981. Perhaps this may look and sound like an autobiography; however, I feel this book may be more aptly categorized as an emotional documentary of the events in my life that helped form the individual I am today.

The house is quiet and our big Italian Mastiff, Lucy, is snoring on her bed in front of the fireplace. Christmas was quiet this year due to all the quarantining and social distancing with the covid virus. Well, quiet is a relative term. We did not have any large family gatherings with extended families; however, we did have Susie's mom, Dolores and our daughter Kendyl move in with us for a couple of months. If anyone was looking for a silver lining to the covid flu outbreak, this was ours. As we know, the special type of interactions and communication one gets from sitting at the dinner table with three generations of ladies for eight weeks creates memories and feelings that will last for the rest of our life. Cooper and his future wife, Deanna, came to visit us for a small holiday gathering with Gramma Dee and Kendyl that was truly special.

My wife, Susie, is sound asleep upstairs. Without Susie I would not be here today. She is my bearing, my light. Her ability to help me see inside myself rather than dwell at the outside influencers, as well as her spiritual guidance and belief in my abilities, has more than once saved me from myself. These pages are as much about what she has endured with me as they are about the stories we have shared together. Honestly, I look forward to experiencing the emotions these stories will unfold over the following months.

Yesterday, New Year's Day, Kendyl and I took the dogs and went for a hike. Kendyl has been living and making her life in New York City since she graduated college; however, since covid, she has been working from home. She decided it would be just as easy to work from home in Santa Cruz, rather than stay cooped up in her Upper East Side apartment. Assuming covid lets up, she will most likely head back to NYC sometime in the next couple months.

Anyway, back to the walk I took with Kendyl. Early New Year's Day we packed both of our dogs, Lucy, and Nico, into the truck and drove down to Nicene Marks Park in Aptos. It had recently rained so the trails were muddy and the mist that hung below the mossy redwood trees was of a completely mystical world. When talking, I tend to go right in with curious and intimate questions. Not everyone is geared to these types of questions, and over the years, these conversations have not always gone so well with our daughter. Sometimes I think I may push a little hard; however, Susie has helped me practice letting up a bit, with the idea that sometimes less is more. The point is, Kendyl and I walked for over an hour through this magical setting and had amazing conversation the entire time.

Amongst other things, we discussed what we might have for goals for this coming year. This led to a conversation about what we think we are good at doing and what it means to be good at something. Somehow, we went down the path of discussing the difference between being born with a particular talent as opposed to practicing something on a regular schedule to become accomplished. She shared with me specifics about what she would like to be doing, her talents, and how she thinks the year will unfold for her. As well, I was discussing the different projects that I

2

am working on and my feeling that it would do me well to author a book about health literacy or some such pharmacy topic.

After a little more discussion, it became evident to me that before I will be able to sit and write about health literacy or other pharmacy topics, first I need to write this book.

***

After writing at least twice weekly for a good 12 months, I found I had plenty of compelling material; however, who was I writing for? Who is my audience?

Do I write just about addiction, or maybe just about pharmacy? My story, in order to be complete, needs to also include my relationship with my wife, Susie. Actually, the more I meditated on the topic, I began to understand that Susie is continually at the center of my story.

Writing a story specifically about addiction, or even more succinct, a story about a pharmacist in the midst of addiction, would not completely tell my story. Throughout the practice of pharmacy over the past four decades, as well as the insidious addictive lifestyle and gracious recovery, my family has been present. My wife, children, parents, brothers and sisters; they are all part of who I am today.

This book is difficult to fit into a particular category. It specifically does not just focus on addiction and recovery; however, the entire book revolves around both of these incredibly huge topics.

As well, the practice of pharmacy has been at the center of my life since the spring of 1981. All the choices that went into deciding why I chose pharmacy school, working my way through college, practicing pharmacy in all types of practice settings. This alone should be ample topic to complete an entire book; however, again, this is only a portion of who I am and how I came to be the person I am today.

Like everyone I have ever met, I come from a family and have a family of my own. Everyone, on some level, can relate to this. Our family, past and present, influence who we become.

More than anything else, my partner in life, who I have been connected to since the fall of 1979, is the center of my story. As you will come to understand throughout these pages.

1

Introduction

Susie and I have developed an incredibly strong emotional thread that weaves our small family together. Certainly, many families must experience this level of connectivity; however, I am sure that many are broken apart for some reason or other and never quite realize the strength in a connected love.

During our early years as a family, we had some troubled times. Throughout these pages I will talk about this and how we worked through the difficulties. Everything we have gone through; all the conversations, laughter, and tears, which have brought us to where we are today. Believe me, this was not an easy process. We all have had opportunities to address situational issues that affected our lives, and we know, as time passes, more discussions will be had. The point is, we are open to healing.

Today we are a healthy and functional family. We all have our way of communicating with each other and it is accompanied with a healthy understanding of how the others will react to our specific level of discussion.

To help place my story in perspective, first I need to take a moment and share where I came from in my early years. Thinking of the joy I experienced during my grade school years nearly brings tears to my eyes, it was an incredibly beautiful time in life.

Thinking back, I remember riding home on the school bus from Quail Hollow elementary school, toward the end of the school year in 3rd grade. The bus is traveling down highway nine through Ben Lomond, heading north just prior to the Tyrolean Inn. Sitting up in the seat we are all looking out the window toward Ben Lomond Park and the river. The picture is clear as day in my brain. The dam had been put in the river that morning and the river was filling up for summertime swimming. Every year, the excitement of the dam being put up was the beginning of the quintessential Ben Lomond summer.

For what seemed like years; however, it was probably from five years old until somewhere in my early teens, I would stay up late on summer nights watching comedy shows with my brother David or one of my friends that was spending the night.

We would sleep in till at least 10am the next morning, then, after a big bowl of Wheaties with sugar or a waffle or some other amazing creation that Mom would make, we would be down at the river playing and swimming. Without describing the entire scene, such as the Little Beach that we hung out on, our excellent wooden boat or the amazing blackberries we would gorge ourselves with toward the end of summer, I mainly would like to convey how it all came together to make me feel.

At the time I did not realize this; however, summertime in Ben Lomond in the late 60's and early 70's was idyllic. We were sequestered into our own little time warp that seemed to hang on forever. This entire amazing life was fully taken for granted; I knew of no other.

My seven older brothers and sisters would come at different times and amaze me with their fantastical worldly wisdom and never-ending stream of boyfriends and girlfriends. The attention they would give me was just soaked up like the sponge that I was, never getting enough but always feeling satisfied.

My time playing with nephews and nieces was constant, always floating on the water, building forts in the back yard and relentless wrestling matches in the sand and weeds.

After dinner, Mom and Dad were always willing to go for an evening paddle in the river on the boat. Mom has a towel ready for me as I crawl back into the boat after the sun has gone down and the mosquitos are ready to dive headlong into my plump flesh. This was normal to me. The feeling that life is at a standstill and will continually be pictured as one ever lasting snapshot in time. Maybe that is why these are called the wonder years?

By the time I had reached ninth grade, all of my seven brothers and sisters had moved out of the house and on with their lives. Well, moved out, yes; however, growing up in a big, loving, and welcoming family, we all know that family is never really gone.

Whether it was a summer break, two weeks between military deployments, in-between houses, or just an extended Christmas holiday; siblings were always coming and going.

On the other hand, I had Mom and Dad completely to myself. Thinking back on it, nearly five decades ago, they were both present, every single day, to talk with me and listen to my dreams of future life. As a teenager I was incredibly fortunate to have both parents front and center in my life, showing up for athletic events, helping me with studies, and supporting me in any way they could.

Being the last of eight children, by the time I came around, both Mom and Dad said they had seen it all. Their practice with me was, it seemed, was to give me as much space as I needed to be a teenager.

As I will get into later in the book, I learned as a freshman in high school how I could drink a couple beers and all of a sudden be awakened to a personality deep down inside of me. My character was transformed into someone who was outgoing, mischievous, flirtatious, and perhaps even a little rebellious.

On the other hand, I was an excellent student, received good grades, and always completed my assignments early. In addition, I worked regular hours, initially washing dishes at a local diner, then, as a freshman in high school, working 20 hours per week at our local grocery store. I was always well funded and never needed to ask my parents for money to go out with my friends or on a date.

Early on in my teenage years I learned how to lie about what I was going to be doing for an evening out. I say this matter-of-factly because that is exactly what I did. I would tell my parents I was going bowling or to the movies, borrow our family car, and proceed to get drunk with three or four of my friends.

Sometime after midnight I would be driving home, through the backroads so there would be less of a chance for police to see me. The car window would be down for the fresh air on my face and my hand covering my eye, so I was not seeing double lanes.

Looking back, I am absolutely and unequivocally positive that it was God's grace allowing me to make it home without injuring myself or someone else.

The next morning Dad would come to wake me up at 7:30 am so we could be out the door by 7:45 and on our way to Sunday mass at St. Michaels Church. I knew I had to get up, wash my face and hold a conversation with my parents. This is how it worked.

My beginning lessons in life taught me that if I do what is expected of me; get good grades in school, perform well at work, maintain some sort of athletic ability, and do my best to communicate well with my elders, well then, I could get away with just about anything I wanted to.

What I am doing here in my teenage years is setting up a pendulum theme that follows me through my 20's and into my early 30's. As the pendulum swings one way, I am gaining positive reinforcement from the people around me, people pleasing. Deep in my core I realized nothing felt quite as nice as hearing how good I was doing from someone I admired. As the pendulum would swing to the other side, I find myself numbing myself as to ward off the ability to feel emotions.

Throughout this tumultuous course I am on, life continues. After working my way through six years of college, I graduate pharmacy school with honors, quickly move into hospital pharmacy management, marry the love of my life, father two lovely children and move through three home purchases, all before the age of 32.

The following pages will share glimpses into what drove my decision process while working my way through college, as well as my inability to appropriately share my emotions during the early years of my professional career. Moreover, I strive to give credit to my wife, Susie, for the faith she had in our family and life together.

Distinctly, I recall sitting in a group session, the first night in a rehab facility in Santa Cruz, listening to other alcoholics describe how they ended up here. Remarkably, although our stories were, in many ways quite different, they were also incredibly similar. This began a lifelong practice of learning and applying the tools necessary to live a sober, honest, and grateful life.

Both our children were under five years old when I came home from 28 days in the drug and alcohol treatment facility. The story of living sober, with family, begins here. Our focus on building a solid foundation, the expansion through the wonder years, and finally, preparing our children to launch into their own lives.

It is my desire to share with you the emotional ride we had as a family working through all these years.

As a pharmacist, I had been granted a second chance for a career. With a new understanding of the tools necessary to live an authentic life, I re-ignited my career as a hospital and community pharmacist. With multiple opportunities to develop clinically oriented programs, I hope to share some of what I have learned while practicing pharmacy for nearly four decades.

It is my sincere hope that while reading these pages of my emotional documentary, you may, on some level, relate to the spiritual, physical, and emotional challenges we face as humans. Our authentic self is within us; however, we all wear masks to define us otherwise. With grace, and a healthy serving of naked vigilance, we may begin to peel away the layers and expose our authentic self.

2

Pre-Pharmacy

The Fall of 1981 saw me off to the University of the Pacific as a pre-pharmacy student. This was it. I was now a freshman in college preparing my way to enter the professional school of pharmacy.

Fortunately, I had qualified for federal and state funding as well as some scholarship money and the incredibly expensive private university was suddenly affordable. Unfortunately, throughout my entire high school career, I had not learned how to properly study.

During high school I had learned, what seemed like, excellent student survival skills. My ability to quickly ascertain exactly what the teacher was looking for helped me graduate high school as an honor student with well above a 3.5 grade point average. After four weeks of college, I abruptly learned that these skills were all but useless in my current situation.

Compared to my years of high school studies, college was difficult, verging on unobtainable. Extensive note taking and time management were foreign tools to me. I can recall sitting at my dormitory desk mid-afternoon on a sunny fall day. My chemistry book opened in front of me with a series of 10 or 12 chemistry word problems I needed to work through. Maybe we had covered the subject in class; however, I could not tell by looking through my notes. Evidently, it was up to me to review the 35-page chapter and figure out how to work through the problems.

After what seemed an eternity, I had managed to maybe work my way through the first problem. I could hear my friends in the hallway, through the open dorm room door, getting ready to head down to the dining hall for dinner.

I had not learned how to be a student. I was completely unaware of a path I could take that would lead me toward becoming a better student. Watching my roommate and other students, I thought I might be able to use some of my old high school skills and get by. Really, the only applicable tools I had at the time were my fake ID so I could buy alcohol for my classmates and a personality that was willing to instigate and participate in mischievous behavior.

One evening, during the Winter of 1980 while I was a junior in high school, I was downstairs in our basement, tuning my skis for an upcoming trip to Tahoe. Dad came down to chat and we had the discussion (again) about what I was going to study in college.

It was gentle, yet directional and filled with intent. He knew I needed a plan; he was encouraging me to develop it before it was directed at me. My thoughts at the time; I wanted an advanced degree without eight years of school, the guarantee of a well-paying position when I graduated, and the option to choose any city in the country to go to. At the time, it was important for me to understand exactly what I would be doing when I graduated. Architecture and photography were interesting; however, I was certain I would need to move wherever the job was located, rather than pick where I wanted to go. The Air Force Academy was toward the top of my list; but the hurdles to overcome seemed too grandiose. Both medicine and law were options; however, first I would need an undergraduate degree, then the professional school. This seemed far too long.

After a month of spreadsheets, pharmacy filtered to the top. University of the Pacific offered a five year Doctor of Pharmacy program that appeared to fit all of my requirements. The plan was to complete two years of pre-pharmacy requirements, then, without an undergraduate degree, enter the professional pharmacy program. The doctorate degree was still an eight semester program; however, it went year-round so it would be complete in three years.

Well now, there I was, the week before Thanksgiving vacation 1981, in complete turmoil. Pre-pharmacy midterms had come and gone and left me with a C- in chemistry and a D in biology. I don't remember ever getting a C in any class in high school, and definitely never a D. I had made up my mind, I was going to let my family know I would be leaving the University of the Pacific at the end of my first semester and moving to South Lake Tahoe to pursue my dream of skiing.

Looking back, it wasn't necessarily about skiing, but rather, I was deathly afraid I would fail out of college and disappoint my parents and family. I hadn't yet realized I was capable of university level academics; however, I was reasonably sure I would excel at the community college in South Lake Tahoe; and yes, the skiing.

Thanksgivings at the Leuck home in Ben Lomond, during the 70's and early 80's, were tremendous gatherings. Mom and Dad were the center and we all gathered to be with them in our big house to celebrate and eat together. My older brothers and sisters had new families and young children. Family and friends would come and go over the holiday; however, Thanksgiving dinner was always a tremendous buffet of everything you could imagine. The adults would mostly all be pushed around the table, and then there were countless others sitting wherever we could throughout the living room.

The story here is not about the grandiose family gatherings at my birth house, but rather, the emotional hurricane I endured, the youngest of eight children, when I let my entire family know I'm dropping out of a fully funded university pharmacy school program to go skiing.

Both Mom and Dad were incredibly supportive. The previous night I had a conversation with them, and as I recall, it went relatively well. I had come prepared with a plan. To their credit, never do I recall my parents directly over riding me with a parental edict. Both Mom and Dad had instilled in me early on the importance of creating a plan of what I wanted to do, evaluating that plan, and then implementing the steps of that plan.

When I was presenting my current plan, to Mom and Dad, of leaving the university and moving to Tahoe, the focus of the conversation centered around my dream to see if I could make some kind of life through skiing. What we did not discuss was my underlying fear that I would most likely fail out of the university before I even got to the pharmacy program and the unbearable amount of disappointment that may cause.

Sometime toward the end of dinner that Thanksgiving Day the plan surfaced as family dinner discussion, and everyone got involved. I remember sitting in a dining room chair in the middle of the living room and all of my brothers and sisters expressing either their disapproval of my decision or their excitement for what was ahead.

Of my seven older brothers and sisters, five of them had graduated college. The thing is, they all took the long way, traveling and working before settling into their chosen field of study. In their opinion, I was the one who was going to be different. What was I thinking? I had been offered a nearly fully funded university education and was going to throw it all away to chase some sort of skiing dream?

During the couple of hours that we talked I stood my ground. My plan was laid out clear and concise. I would get an apartment in Tahoe with some of my friends, attend Lake Tahoe Community College as a full-time student, get part time work, and ski as much as I could. What we didn't discuss was my underlying fear of disappointing them through my misguided understanding of how to be a student.

Had I voiced my true concern about my lack of preparedness for college life, I am certain that every one of my siblings would have stepped forward with support and love. They had all been through difficult situations in their life and I now know that each one of them carries wisdom beyond belief.

Unfortunately for me, at that point in my life, my entire being was focused on gaining approval, not disappointing. At the time, the disappointment endured for leaving the university and moving to Tahoe was far less than the potential disappointment failing out of the pre-pharmacy program would have caused.

About three weeks before school was out, I was sitting in my dorm room with some friends drinking beers on a Friday night, as usual. Someone brought up the idea that we should go to Jack-in-the-Box and grab some food. Great idea! As we were walking down the hall, I noticed the multi-purpose room at the end of the hall was full of all the kids in my hall. I was initially concerned that we were missing a hall meeting. We walked in, all quiet like, and I sat on the floor against the wall to listen in. No one was talking and everyone was looking at me. I leaned forward and looked up at a banner they had put on the wall which read, "We'll Miss You Steve, Good Luck". The part that got me was that in a short 3-month time, I had made some great friends. I had never had to make friends before. I went to kinder-garden with the same group I graduated high school with. In my short stint at UOP, I had made some close friends and, surprisingly, I was incredibly sad that last week of school.

Soon enough I was packing up my belongings from the University of Pacific, saying goodbye to my college friends, and moving myself home. Christmas was just around the corner, and I was focused on assuring my plan was in place for the move to Tahoe.

Yes, this was an incredibly challenging time in my life, and yes, I wasn't completely honest with myself or my family with regards to my emotions or motives; however, I did learn an incredibly valuable lifelong lesson during the last couple months of 1981. When I take time to create a plan, follow through completely on all aspects of that plan, more often than not, I get exactly what I planned for.

3

One School at a Time

Throughout the next five and one-half years, I became the quintessential college student. My grades slowly increased with a consistent margin. Concentrated involvement and participation in collegiate and extracurricular activities grew on a steady and positive trend line. Principally, as time passed, the fear of failing became a distant memory as my self-assured confidence began to grow stronger every single day.

Moving to Tahoe gave me the outward feeling that I was making it on my own. Through a series of phone interviews, I had secured a lease in a two bedroom apartment for myself and three friends to move into. The lease was in my name, and I had coordinated all the specifics surrounding its acquisition. As well, I had organized our utilities and managed to have the heat, electricity, water, and phone all connected by the day we moved in on the day after Christmas, 1982.

Our first two weeks in Tahoe was somewhat of a vacation for myself and my three new roommates. School had not yet started, and no one had a job yet, so it was pretty much game-on. We arrived and unpacked the day after Christmas, and the day after that the biggest snowstorm of the year hit. Many of our friends had arrived for vacation, and good thing they were already there because highway 50, in and out of Tahoe, closed down for nearly a week.

Our road was a dead-end road, so it was low priority as far as plowing goes. Fortunately, we could walk to a liquor store, and we had an apartment full of friends. Soon enough the snowplow made it down our little road, firing snow out from under the blade, forming a nice ledge on the side of the road about five feet tall. With time on our hands, we came up with a plan. First, we took about 60 minutes to dig out my little Honda Civic, which had been completely buried by the storm.

Next, we pulled the car out onto our little road and procured about a 30-foot-long rope which we secured to the back bumper. With my boots and skis on, my friend drove my little Honda up and down the road with me skiing behind. After we all had turns, we then built a ramp on the side of the road, going up the ledge. Coming down the road at a quick clip, I was slaloming back and forth, spraying the fresh powder like I was water skiing. Zig zagging back and forth, I took one last zag and dropped the rope as I went hurling toward the five foot ramp. Launching, I traveled through the air until I came crashing down into shoulder deep powder.

Our first day of class at Lake Tahoe Community College was definitely a memorable experience. Us four San Lorenzo Valley boys, not being used to living in the snow, did not have any knowledge of the different school rules, like perhaps if there is three feet of fresh snow on the road school may be canceled for the day. School was about two miles away and my friend and I were on the road to class an hour before class time.

We are on highway 50, driving in the one lane that was open, watching the snow in the center of the road grow to about a six foot wall. As we get to school, we plow through the break in the wall and maintain enough speed to push over the hump of snow blocking the parking lot entrance. Here we are, stuck in the middle of an unplowed parking lot, and no one else at school.

We desperately failed at our attempts to push the snow out of the way to give the chains something to grip onto besides powder snow. Now, directly behind us, comes a snowplow, with the driver upset with us because we are blocking his way. I jokingly holler at him to shove us out of the lot. That is all it took; he was then heading directly toward the back of my car. We scramble to get inside the car just before the tractor comes pushing up against the back of the Honda and then propels us twenty feet through the lot with snow coming up over the front of the car. We really were not sure if we should thank him or be upset at him for breaking one of my back tail lights and denting my bumper. I guess it was better than being buried in the middle of the lot.

Fortunately I had two strong reasons to stay in school. First, I would continue to be covered under my parents' health insurance until I was 23 years old as long as I was in school. Secondly, due to the fact Dad was retired and Mom was on disability, as long as I maintained my status as a full-time student, I would receive a check from the government for $320 per month. This was fantastic. It is crazy thinking about it in today's terms; however, this was plenty of money to cover my rent, utilities, food, and tuition at Lake Tahoe Community College. This was a short-lived benefit and was canceled with the new administration; however, it sure made a difference during the winter and spring of 1982.

During my six months in Tahoe, I managed to be hired onto, and quit, six part time jobs. Everything from pizza delivery, bag boy, dish washer, hotel cleaner and ski lift operator; my work ethic was that of a manipulator. When I needed a little extra spending money, I realized, with smart words and positive assurance, I could easily be hired.

After a few weeks, some dark corner of my personality had convinced me it was totally fine to get my paycheck, and then just not show up for my next shift. This was still early on in my adult career development; however, the supply of endorphins generated from taking that last check, knowing I had no plans of returning for my next scheduled workday, was an emotion I was getting used to. As well, the ease at which I was able to get another job boosted my self confidence in a tremendously inappropriate way.

Skiing during the winter of 1982 was exciting, reckless, fast, often uncoordinated, and most often daily. More often than not, I was under the influence of alcohol or pot while I was on the way to, on or coming home from the mountain. Over the past 40 years it has been easy for me to romanticize and glamorize this season, but in reality, it was not romantic or glamorous. More concisely, it was emotionally dark, dangerous, and commonly deceitful.

Do not misunderstand me, I became a well-qualified skier this year. My abilities and skills grew exponentially chasing hot shots around the mountain and down the moguls, but my illicit and mischievous behavior was far from graceful.

My finances were such that I did not have any money left over for ski passes, being that any residual income was frequently spent on alcohol, pot, and on the rare occasion, cocaine. To ski, I would steal my way onto the mountain with second hand tickets. The grift was, I would show up to the mountain at about 11am and wait in the parking lot for someone coming back to their car. As I approach them, I would ask if I could clip off their ticket and put it to use for the rest of the day. Most of the time, the first person I asked would say yes. If they put up any kind of resistance, I would quickly move on, not bothering to engage them any further. Always, a willing individual would come along. After using my wire cutters to clip off their ticket, I would spray chemicals on the back of the pass, which allowed me to peel it apart and place it on a new hanger on my jacket. Rarely was I not on the chairlift by noon.

The practice of clipping tickets was not new to ski areas. The resorts understood this happened and had patrol in the parking lot looking to catch the criminals in the act and have them detained or arrested. During my time in Tahoe, I was aware of a few of my acquaintances who got caught. My trouble was, I was good at it. Somehow, I had a clear sense of situational awareness which allowed me to make it through the season without incident. Once again, this only added to my misguided sense of self-worth.

Just as I had predicted, school was easy. The tools I had used in high school to determine what was necessary to get good grades totally applied here. With little effort I was able to excel in class. In addition, I was able to schedule my classes either in the morning or at night so as not to interfere with my daily afternoon ski schedule.

One of my required classes was U.S. History. This professor was retired from the University of California Santa Barbara and had moved up to Tahoe for his retirement, and a little bit of teaching. He was an excellent instructor, engaging and thoughtful in his conversations, but more than that, he carried with him a message that he cared for the outcome of his students. During one of his evening classes, mid spring semester, he got off on a tangent discussing what we were all doing in Tahoe. His tone was harsh, yet compelling. He went on to ask us how we planned on living anything like the life we had grown up with. He was referring to the idea that we grew up in a nice home, food in the kitchen and two cars in the driveway. He wanted to know when we were planning to grow up and take responsibility for our own life. What were our plans and how were we going to make them happen?

This was an indelible moment in my life, and it completely changed my trajectory. That evening I realized I was ready to start over, do my pre-pharmacy requirements, and continue my path to pharmacy school. Perhaps it was the ill acquired self-confidence I had gained through my exploits in Tahoe, or maybe a higher power steering me in a different direction during a moment of receptiveness; regardless, the professor had voiced his concerns and I had begun creating a plan.

Of course, after moving home for summer I could have stayed and performed my studies at the local community college. Perhaps that would have been the financially prudent move on my part; however, my plan took me elsewhere. To save money, I left my car in Ben Lomond and found myself in a U-Haul heading to San Diego State University during the last days of our 1982 summer.

My plan included retaking first year chemistry and biology over from the start. This was my second chance at making a grade, and I knew I needed to make it work. My six months in Tahoe had given me the self-assuredness and confidence I required to make it work, now I just needed to learn how to study.

20

My good friend Brad was in his second year at SDSU and had invited me to move in with him and a couple of his friends in an off-campus apartment. Not far from school, I would ride my bicycle the mile and a half to campus every morning. Coming back home midafternoon that first week of school I noticed something a bit odd. Brad would be in his room, at his desk, with his books open working on whatever needed to be done.

Evidently, this is the simple tool necessary to pass classes. I needed to follow Brad's lead and sit at my desk for three or four hours every afternoon and get the day's work done. As if a lightning bolt had burst through the clouds and shot me in the head, I had cracked the code. College classes dump an incredible amount of information onto students. After living through six years of college, I am convinced that four hours solid study, at least six days per week, is more than adequate to learn the material and pass classes with decent grades.

With an idea that I needed to learn what it meant to work in a pharmacy, I applied for a clerk position at a medical clinic pharmacy that just happened to be halfway between our apartment and school. After stopping by the store, a couple times and applying every bit of over-confident 18-year-old allure I possessed, I was offered a job.

This was my first introduction to working in a pharmacy, and I loved it. Not only was the pharmacist witty and smart, but he also carried with him a deep understanding and compassion for every patient that walked into the little clinic pharmacy. His ability to retrieve, what seemed to be out of thin air, the constant answers to questions from the physicians in the clinic was awe inspiring.

San Diego taught me how to pay attention in class, study and manage my time. On the other hand, as simple as it sounds, it is still hard work. Emotionally, I found myself wanting to check out and live without responsibility. As a tool, I found that pot, which was incredibly available everywhere, did an amazing job of helping me temporarily check out. The dissociative feeling was like a temporary vacation from life. Regrettably, two hours later I was sleepy and incredibly non-productive.

Much to my astonishment, I soon found a solution that would carry me through the next five years.

One afternoon, rather than sit and listen to music with my roomies after smoking pot, I put on my running shoes, got my Walkman, and headed out for a run. Feeling the music resonate through my neural pathways I glided effortlessly down the sidewalks of San Diego, through the university campus, down suburban streets, making my way back to the apartment six miles later. Not only did I feel as if I had just been on a weeklong emotional vacation, but my body also felt strong and alive. I was refreshed, awake, clear headed and ready to step right back into the study-work-school cycle.

Confident and ready to work my way back to the University of the Pacific, I finished my year at San Diego and headed back home for the summer. Maintaining momentum, I elected to take a full years' worth of organic chemistry this summer at the University of California in Santa Cruz. Now realizing I do my best work when my schedule is full, I was at a lecture and lab five days per week in Santa Cruz, staying at my sister's house in her back cabin to minimize study distractions.

On the weekend I would head back up to Ben Lomond and stay with Mom and Dad and work both days at Ben Lomond Super grocery store. Memories of late weekend dinners on the back porch with Mom and Dad echo through my heart. Both were healthy that summer, walking and working in the yard. Sharing my hopes and dreams while listening to their stories of life while relaxing on the back porch will resonate with me forever.

The emotional support from parents is something I took for granted at this time in my life. Over the past four decades I have looked back on this summer from time to time with warmth and fondness. This time I had with my parents, feeling as if I was almost an adult, having real-life conversations with them, helped secure my commitment to fully completing my pharmacy school education.

Fall of 1983 saw me resuming my studies at the University of the Pacific; however, this time I was entering the school on academic probation. Remember, just 20 months ago I had left UOP for fear of failing. Interestingly, academic probation did not seem to concern me. Having cracked-the-code to college studying, the thought of failing out of any class was a distant, if not forgotten, fear.

Over the past two years, I had learned a few important lessons. From my first semester at UOP, I had learned that, even if my motives may not be entirely honest, I had the skill set within me to create a plan, put it into action, and make something happen. Next, through my time in Tahoe, I had gained an inappropriately elevated level of self-esteem, with the underlying thought that my mischievous behavior could rarely, if ever, be called into question. Thankfully, in San Diego I had discovered the secret to successful studying; time and focus. Finally, moving back to Santa Cruz for the summer I was able to finally comprehend the magnificent power of time management, unlocking the power of each and every hour.

Gathering all these tools together and holding them in my back pocket I begin my years at UOP.

As the semesters on campus passed, I became integrally involved with campus activities, intramural athletics, fraternity life, pharmacy intern jobs and student-pharmacy organization opportunities. Immersing myself in the college lifestyle brought opportunities for involvement such as Mr. April on the Men of Pacific calendar, student adviser to incoming freshmen, member of the 84-85 homecoming court, and California Society of Hospital Pharmacists student of the year.

On the one hand, participation in the college lifestyle greatly increased my ability to communicate; however, on the other hand, I was increasingly looking for angles to up my status in the eyes of my peers. I was a friend to many; however, perhaps not the most genuine or authentic individual.

When I first came back to UOP I had taken an elective class on interpersonal communication. This taught me the tools of how to listen and engage an individual on their level. It was quite effective, and people love to share when they have someone who will listen. The thing is, I had not learned how to authentically share back. I had the stories of where I had been and what I had done, but never was I able to share how I was feeling.

Unlike most schools, UOP has an accelerated program. Assuming the applicant has met all the undergraduate requirements, an undergraduate degree was not necessarily required. Then, beginning with the first semester, the pharmacy student completes six semesters of course work and two semesters of clinical rotations in three fun-packed years, graduating with their doctorate degree in pharmacy.

Before I knew it, four years had passed, and I had moved myself from academic probation to the deans' honor roll. As if the goddess Hygeia, herself, had come down and anointed me from the bowl of good health, I was ready to begin my practice of pharmacy.

My audience had changed. For years, growing up and working my way through high school, I had sought the approval of my parents as well as my brothers and sisters. Through college, this approval seeking behavior grew, as I performed for fellow students and my instructors at every opportunity.

As I mentioned back in the introduction, this pendulum theme is beginning to grow. The more I perform in college, the higher the approval bar moves, and the higher the pendulum swings. Correspondingly, as the pendulum swings back the other way it also swings higher.

Unconsciously searching for new ways to anesthetize my emotions, I find my running has increased as well as my pot smoking. In addition, on weekends and holidays, it was not uncommon to be drinking by 10am.

So here I am, a high performing pharmacy student, graduating with a Doctorate in Pharmacy, ready to take the state board of pharmacy examination, who's only tools to manage emotions are alcohol, marijuana, and exercise.

4

Coming Home

It had been about 12 months since I graduated pharmacy school and I was living in a home with a pharmacy school friend in the Seabright area of Santa Cruz, just a couple blocks behind the Seabright Brewery. My good friend had been a year in front of me through pharmacy school and was settling in quite nicely to the Santa Cruz lifestyle. In the spring of 1988, he was in the process of purchasing a new home just two blocks back from Castle Beach. It was my good fortune that he had a room for rent at just the same time I had come back into town and needed a place of my own to stay.

Directly after college I had moved home to study for the state pharmacy board examination. Fortunately, Mom and Dad still lived in Ben Lomond and had plenty of room for me to come stay. Their house was always open to their children. The upstairs bedroom was transformed into a study hall and for four fast weeks I lived inside of all the books I had been studying the last eight semesters. To help my situation, a seasoned local pharmacist graciously hired me at the local drug store to work as a pharmacy intern. In my opinion, nothing better prepares a young mind for a pharmacy examination like practical experience. More than just working in the pharmacy as an intern, I would evaluate every medication bottle I touched to be certain I knew all of the data and specifics. By the end of each day, I would go home to my study hall with my pockets full of package inserts to review and quiz myself with.

The time came for the test, and I traveled to Southern California for a weekend. State examination boards like this are a daunting experience. The examination consisted of eight separate tests, each one being two hours long. Before 2004, California had its own pharmacy examination. All of the other states participated in a national exam which would allow for license reciprocation from one state to another, but not California. If someone wanted to practice pharmacy in California, they had to take and pass the state's own specific examination. Supposedly, the state's three pharmacy schools were the best equipped in the country to prepare an individual for said exam. Hundreds of graduates, as well as hundreds of pharmacists from other states wanting to practice pharmacy in California would congregate in this enormous room. Test monitors would stand at every other table to assure no one would be looking at others for help. In any given year, only 40-50% of the test takers would pass the examination. In all my years of studying and test taking, nothing compares to the anxiety and tension surrounding this experience. After completion of the test, it was nearly three months before we received our results letter; I am happy to say I passed with 87%.

Exactly seven days later I was sitting in a similar room in Boston taking the Massachusetts state board of pharmacy examination. Although the room and students felt familiar, the nature of the examination couldn't have been more different. It wouldn't be appropriate of me to say the exam was simple; however, because I had prepared so intensely for the difficult California examination, the Massachusetts test felt like a basic review of my memory.

Many of my friends from pharmacy school were in a position where they could travel after graduation. My situation was a little different in that I needed to prepare for the upcoming student loans that would need to begin payment six months after graduation. My goal was to see a bit of an unknown world while still practicing pharmacy, and through a series of events, I chose Boston. The city, with such a deep historical background, was seen through a runner's eyes. My days off were spent on long runs, getting lost through Beacon Hill, the Back Bay, the North End, and the long trails along the Charles River.

My first pharmacist job as a licensed practitioner was in Everett, Massachusetts, just a short subway ride outside of Boston. Osco Pharmacy was a local chain store at the time. Twelve-hour shifts, no breaks, no computers, and relatively little help in the store led me to question why I decided to move into this profession in the first place. Where was the clinical practice of visiting with patients, consulting physicians and being on the care team we had all talked about in pharmacy school. By October 1987, four months after arriving in Boston, I was ready to leave. Chain pharmacy practice was not for me; besides, I missed Santa Cruz.

The late 80's and early 90's was a time of growth and expansion in the pharmacy world. Jobs for pharmacists were everywhere. After a couple of phone calls to the hospitals in Santa Cruz, I promptly had a position lined up as a staff pharmacist at Community Hospital of Santa Cruz and was scheduled to start just prior to Christmas. Once again, I recall getting off the airplane in San Francisco with Mom and Dad waiting for me. Graciously, they welcomed me back into their home. My study hall from a few months earlier was still empty upstairs so that became my bedroom for the near future. I assured them it would only be temporary until I found my own place to stay; however, they were quick to let me know they were happy to have me home and that I could stay as long as I liked.

In our twenties, we're doing our best to go out and make it in the world. We launch; however, it is so incredibly wonderful to have parents that understand it's just fine to come back to home, re-group, and then launch again. As I get older, I realize that many young adults don't get this opportunity to come back home when they need to gather themselves before their next launch. Mom and Dad created an environment of hope and optimism and staying with them was always regenerative. As a child I had seen my brothers and sisters come and go, never quite realizing what they were doing; however, always seeing that Mom and Dad encouraged them to come home and then were incredibly supportive of them when they left. These are the exact same feelings I got from them when it was my turn.

When I move into a space, it is always important for me to take some time and make it feel like it is my home. Some folks are able to just slip right in, not change a thing, and call it their space. My life has always been a little different than that. I recall when I was in elementary school, I would go to great lengths to decorate my room. Posters on the wall, my hot wheel collection lined up on my shelves, and my model airplanes painstakingly hung from the ceiling, so it looked like they were dive bombing each other.

This time was no different. My study hall had been the back upstairs portion of the house, so I took it over this time creating my own comfortable loft space. Fresh paint, shelves, a newly purchased stereo system and some well-appointed skiing posters helped create a comfortable space. If I close my eyes, I can still hear the wintertime rush of the San Lorenzo River out the back window. Our house in Ben Lomond was far from a new fancy home; however, it was the quintessential Santa Cruz Mountain home, with a huge back yard and amazing river frontage.

Over the next couple months, I settled into a regular routine of work and exercise. The Community Hospital of Santa Cruz was perfect. Participating in a small community hospital that appreciated and encouraged the pharmacist to be up on the floor, interacting with the nursing staff and helping to resolve medication issues. I can remember feeling like I had found my type of work, this was going to be what I did.

As well, I continued to run and bicycle. Regularly I would work from noon until 9pm, so that left the morning wide open for adventure. It was not uncommon for me to get up, have a cup of coffee, and then be off on a two hour bicycle or running adventure through the San Lorenzo Valley somewhere. This was the middle of winter, 1988, and I had one favorite bike ride I really enjoyed. During this time, the more rain, the better. I would ride toward Felton on highway nine and peddle up behind the high school onto the Fall Creek trail. Following the trail around I would come out at the end of Fall Creek Road and then head back home. By time I would get home, my bike and quite often me, would be covered from head to toe in mud. After a quick hose to both me and the bike, I would take a hot shower, get some breakfast, and head off to work in Santa Cruz.

The time I spent with Mom and Dad during this time was wonderful. We would have lovely conversations over dinner, talk about why we are here on this planet, what the meaning of life is and all sorts of deep and happy thoughts. Looking back on it I can tell they were just enjoying the time, knowing full well that in short order I would be leaving again. As a young professional, I wasn't necessarily thinking about any disruption in their life; however, I am sure they needed to make some adjustments to have me in the house with them again.

After about three months of this my friend let me know that he was purchasing a house in Santa Cruz and could use a roommate. This was the perfect opportunity for me to get back out on my own. Dana had purchased a small home about three blocks behind Seabright Brewery. The house was pretty much brand new; however, it was tiny. Downstairs was a quaint little kitchen and living room with an office off the back and upstairs were two bedrooms.

So, here I am, packing up my little 1976 Honda Civic, once again, and leaving home. The trip was only about 10 miles or so from Ben Lomond down to this little Santa Cruz house just up above the Boardwalk train trestle; however, I believe Mom and Dad realized this was the last time I would be living with them. The departure from Ben Lomond was not filled with tears like it was in 1981 when I left for Stockton or even nine months ago when I left for Boston; instead, it had a sense of completion. The sense was that I had grown into my profession and needed to be living on my own.

Now, back to where this section first started, it's been 12 months since graduation from pharmacy school and I'm living with my good friend in a real-life home just a few blocks from the beach in Santa Cruz. At 24 years old, I feel like I have worked my way into an amazing life. My work is only two miles away, the ocean is a 10-minute walk down the road, and downtown Santa Cruz is just a short bike ride down the hill. Most importantly, the love of my life, Susie, lives three houses back from the beach on 25th avenue, just a simple 15-minute bike ride from my new home.

5

Summer of 88

.

If I am not mistaken, it was the Fall of 1979 that Susie and I first met. Susie was a 14-year-old freshman and I was soon to be 16 years old. For the next two years Susie and I dated on and off. The memories I have of Susie during those two years are absolutely wonderful. Her natural and unpretentious beauty was evident each and every day. Unfortunately, my inability to communicate how I was feeling kept me from committing to a steady relationship during my early years. We really had great times dating, laughing, and getting to know each other but importantly, a spark had been started.

For six years I was away at college. During summers and breaks I would come back to Santa Cruz and quickly look up old friends. Quite often I would call Susie and see how she was doing. In my humble opinion, it was during these visits that Susie and I really began to communicate and share our feelings with each other. Don't get me wrong, Susie wasn't sitting around waiting for me to show up. She was on her own early in her life. Just after she graduated high school her parents moved out of town and Susie decided to stay in Santa Cruz. On her own, at 18 years old, she had an apartment and was working full time paying her own way. When I would come back home for break, I would give her a ring on the phone just to talk and see how she was doing. If her schedule permitted, we might get a bite to eat or catch a movie. She may have been seeing someone else at the time, or maybe I may have been seeing someone else back at college, we never really pressed the issue with each other. As far as we were concerned, we were just two old friends catching up with each other.

When I moved back home after being in Boston, I found myself thinking about Susie, wondering how she was doing with her life. One afternoon I called the clinic where she had worked. The staff assured me that she still worked there; however, she was not working today, and no, they would not give me her phone number. Interestingly, they did offer to give me her mailing address. At home I had been going through a box of old letters that I had kept in the upstairs of the Ben Lomond house. There was this one beautiful card that Susie had sent me a few years back. At this moment I can't remember exactly what it said, however, the sentiment had to do with friends leaving and returning and our hearts always being open to the amazing and special individuals in our life.

Having romantic thoughts, I put the card in an envelope along with a little note that I would like to get together and mailed it off to her. After a couple phone conversations, I found myself sitting on her front stoop waiting for her to come home from work for our first date.

She stepped out of her maroon 1985 5.0L V8 five speed Ford Mustang wearing this lovely short jean skirt and white blouse. Her blonde hair past her shoulders and professional style was breathtaking. Of course, she went on to apologize for keeping me waiting while she was with some of her friends for an after work get together and time got away from her; however, none of that mattered to me at this point.

It was early Spring of 1988, and I was still living at my parents' house in Ben Lomond. Susie's house was near the beach on 25th avenue and the sun hadn't gone down yet, but dusk was coming. I don't believe I was wearing a jacket, and Susie wasn't either when she got out of her car. I think I had knocked on her door and met one of her roommates, who said it would be just fine if I wanted to wait on the front stoop and that Susie should be home any minute.

What an incredibly wonderful date. For what seemed like hours we shared stories over dinner. Sharing our adventures on how we had worked our way through life over the past seven years all leading up to this night. I'm not trying to make this sound like some melodramatic love story; however, when I give myself the opportunity to look back on this particular date from where I sit right now, all the stars were in alignment. Really, could it get any more romantic? I've been going to college and working for seven years. Susie graduated high school, moved out on her own, and has created a self-supporting life for herself here in Santa Cruz. Both of us are not currently dating anyone else. We've gone on dates with each other now and again over the past seven years; however, this is different. Yes, I'd say the stars aligned for us that night.

Dinner was lovely at Margaretville in the Capitola Village. We followed it with a hand-in-hand stroll down the esplanade. Tonight, I can close my eyes and still hear the dance music from the Edgewater Café and smell the pesto and pepperoni from Pizza My Heart. Blossoming romance is a quintessential emotion we can all relate to. Feeling the amazing tingle on my skin as she squeezes my hand, touching the curve of her back and gently letting my hand rest there. We walked down one of the dark sidewalk alleys between two of the restaurants to a small deck overlooking Capitola Beach and the Monterey Bay. From our spot we could see the lights on a few boats anchored not far off the Capitola Beach as well as the lights of the restaurant on the end of the Capitola wharf. I didn't completely realize this at the time, but right there, at that point, I fell for Susie.

The Spring and Summer of 1988 was amazing. Over the next few months, we got to know each other, going on dates, walks, swimming in the ocean, barbequing with friends, and just hanging out with each other. Regularly I would work at the hospital until 9pm. Sometimes, when I would get home to my house in Seabright, I would get a bite to eat, change, and then get on my cruiser and ride over to Susie's house. The foggy evening rides were wet on my face with the taste of salt. My ride took me past the Seabright Brewery, across the Santa Cruz Harbor bridge, down past the harbor entrance and around the Twin-Lakes beach big curve, following East Cliff with a right turn at 17th avenue, past the Villa Maria Del Mar nuns' home, down the hill and up the other side to

25th avenue. Turn right onto 25th and then just a couple houses on the right.

Susie had a little cassette player in her room, like the ones we used to use in elementary school to play school stuff on. You know, the flat ones with the buttons all across the front. She introduced me that summer to music like INXS, Eddie Brickell, and I think her favorite at the time, the Eurythmics. The sound of a song from any of these bands brings me back to that time and space in a heartbeat. Susie needed to start work early at the Scotts Valley Medical Clinic, so she was always up early which had me up and out the door for another foggy bike ride. By no means was this a nightly event; however, over the Summer we definitely had a spark of love, and we really enjoyed each other's company.

One of our dates was a bike ride from Susie's house on 25th down to Capitola for ice cream. Daring as she is, she agreed to ride double with me on my cruiser. I absolutely love that Susie trusted me on my bicycle with her. I would straddle the bike with one foot on the peddle. Susie would then crawl onto the seat, with her legs just hanging out in the air. She would grip my back side, as I peddled, and we would race down the road. From 25th down to Capitola Village is at least two miles and I know we did this more than once without incident.

Another evening in the middle of Summer I somehow talked Susie into camping on the beach just down from her house. Way after dark we packed up our sleeping bags and climbed down the rocks to the sand. The beach is thin along this portion of the coast, so it is not an area that is patrolled by the beach ranger patrol in their trucks. My feeling is, in 1988 the beaches and Santa Cruz as a whole felt much safer and we really didn't think anything of it. Amazingly, looking out over the smokestacks at Moss Landing, we saw the biggest shooting star we have ever seen.

As was the case when I was younger, I was still having a difficult time expressing how I felt. Yes, I had become a much more fluent communicator and was able to carry on a wonderful interpersonal conversation; however, my ability to be vulnerable was poor. I know I felt love coming from within my heart and I could lovingly feel it from Susie. The trouble was, I didn't know how to express this to her in words.

6

Saying Goodbye

As happened regularly that summer, one evening late in July I was out with friends at the Catalyst in downtown Santa Cruz listening to a local band. I can't recall exactly who all was there that evening, or which band was playing; however, I do remember running into an old high school friend who had gone to college to become a nurse. She was down in Santa Cruz on vacation from her new home up in Mt. Shasta where she practiced as an intensive care unit nurse at Mercy Medical Center.

We talked for a while about the mountains surrounding Mt. Shasta, bike riding, and yes of course, skiing. As well we discussed what it was like for her working in the hospital in Mt. Shasta. She explained that Mercy Mt. Shasta was a small hospital, about 20 beds and a four bed ICU. She told me the pharmacy was looking for an additional pharmacist to add to their staff and encouraged me to apply. Sometime within the next couple days I was on the phone calling the hospital and had lined up an interview within the next couple weeks.

Here's the thing, life was great in Santa Cruz. My living arrangements were above par, my employment was booming, and my relationship with Susie was blossoming beyond expectations. Unfortunately for others in my life, my ability to communicate my feelings was lacking and my motivations were relatively self-serving.

I was a dreamer, always have been, always will be. The dream of living and working where I could ski all winter right out my back door had been sitting in my pocket ever since I left South Lake Tahoe the spring of 1982. The thought of looking into pharmacist positions in Tahoe or Colorado, Wyoming or Montana didn't even cross my mind. Mt. Shasta had entered the picture and the dream of living in this small mountain town with its big mountain and upstart ski area was on.

Remembering the days from Tahoe and the winter of 81/82 blinded me from any other ideas. Reminiscing on the less-than-optimal housing arrangements I had in Tahoe as well as the inability to afford ski lift tickets had me thinking about what it would be like in Mt. Shasta. Contemplating how cool it would be to be living in a real home, driving a 4-wheel drive truck in the snow, and being able to ski on every day off kept me laser focused on this new mission.

Within a couple weeks I was on the road to Mt. Shasta for an interview. The top was off my Scout, my mountain bike was in the back, and I was driving up I-5 with the sun glaring down on my sunglasses. The interview went swimmingly, and I was offered the job on the spot. I'm not certain, but most likely I accepted the job on the spot as well. The next day I went on a mountain bike ride with my nurse friend and a group of fellow outdoor enthusiasts for miles down the Pacific Crest Trail. This amazing little mountain town nestled in the shadow of Mt. Shasta was sure to be my new home.

Soon after I got back to Santa Cruz from my Mt. Shasta trip, I had a conversation with my supervisor at Community Hospital. She was accepting of my decision; however, she was clear to state that at some point in my pharmacy career I will need to settle down and keep the same job for a couple of years. She made it clear that if I was to continue to change jobs on an annual basis, my unreliability would quickly catch up to me. That is a message that has stuck with me to this day, and as I'll explain later, I was employed with the same institution for just over 32 years.

Susie and I had been for a walk down on Castle beach. Through a series of sentences that must have sounded nonsensical I described to Susie that I had accepted a job in Mt. Shasta and would be moving north in a couple weeks. This wasn't necessarily a conversation that I was putting forth to get her input on, I was just letting her know this was what I was doing. Even just writing this, I find it hard to imagine how insensitive I was to our relationship.

As well as I can recall, I believe I had an idea that I would move to Mt. Shasta, get settled in a house, and then Susie would come up and move in with me. I feel like I had this all arranged in my head; however, I had not taken the time to adequately express the entire scenario to Susie.

With tears and love we agreed to continue our relationship. Neither of us were sure of how the next few months would work; however, we both agreed we wanted to try. Susie agreed to consider the idea that after I got settled, she would come visit, and we would discuss what moving in together would look like.

Susie and I have both tried to remember when it was that we both said I Love You to each other. Neither of us are able to recall the specifics; however, emotionally, I am certain it was that night.

7

Launching

Of course, Mom and Dad were excited for me. They were just thrilled that I had graduated college and had a profession where I could go just about anywhere I wanted to and get a well-paying, satisfying professional job. During this period I was up in Ben Lomond, visiting and preparing for my move. Next door, in the big green house, there happened to be a trailer in the yard for sale. Not just any trailer, this was an early model Chevy pickup truck bed welded and bolted to an incredibly sturdy trailer chassis. Not the prettiest trailer I have ever seen; however, one of the most functional hauling trailers on this planet. It just so happened that I had recently sold my 1976 Honda Civic for $250 to one of my friends at the Santa Cruz Community hospital. Wonderfully, the trailer was for sale for $250. This was an even trade for me, perfect.

As I think back on the move from Santa Cruz to Mt. Shasta, I wonder what I could have possibly needed a trailer for. Yes, I was moving 400 miles away to start my life in a new town; however, what could I have possibly owned that needed a trailer? Regardless, I do remember packing both my Scout as well as the trailer to the top. I am sure I must have packed a bed and a chair or two, skis, exercise machine, bicycle, stereo, records, and boxes. This was me leaving Ben Lomond. Anything from the house that I had collected over the years went in boxes and came with me including books that I had collected, my hot wheel collection and of course a toolbox full of functional items Dad helped me pick out from the basement.

My roommate in Santa Cruz was sad to see me go. We had gotten to know each other well over the course of the last few months, and to this day I don't think we have seen each other more than twice over the past four decades. On the other hand, he was engaged to be married within the next couple months so my imminent departure from his home had already been slated. Me leaving gave him and his fiancé an opportunity to prepare the house with all the comforts a couple of newlyweds should have in a new home.

Leaving Ben Lomond this time doesn't register in my memory the same way it did the previous times I had loaded up and left. I know my truck and trailer were packed tight, but it doesn't register as that significant of a departure. Maybe it was because I had already left home and dealt with those emotions when I moved to Santa Cruz six months earlier. As I sit here and write this, I can picture myself driving around the sharp freeway onramp in Scotts Valley, just passing by the Scotts Valley Medical Clinic where Susie was working. I knew we would be together again, and I knew Susie loved me.

The road to Mt. Shasta from Santa Cruz, in a 1973 truck, pulling a pickup truck bed trailer, in the heat of September is a long drive. After you get past the Nut Tree and onto I-5 heading north, the road just feels like it goes on forever. Little towns followed by rest stops with two trees for shade are what I see for the next three hours. Today I realize three hours is really not that long of a time; however, at 24 years old, the road seemed to never end. Soon the signs for Red Bluff and Redding start to appear. As I look North, I can see the faint outline of this tremendous mountain. As Redding gets closer the mountain outline begins to gain visual clarity and I realize within the next two hours I will be parking at the base of that mountain, creating my new home.

Here's the thing, I was packed up and moving to Mt. Shasta to start a new job, and I didn't yet have any idea where I was going to live. My nursing friend who had originally told me about the position had arranged for me to stay at the place she was renting for a couple days, but I needed to find a place quickly. Interestingly, this did not bother me one bit. It's difficult for me to imagine today moving to a new town with all my worldly belongings and not preemptively having arranged my housing. My concern was very little. Somehow, I knew it would work out just fine. When I got to Mt. Shasta, I had about 10 days before I needed to start work, so I knew I would be set up somewhere in plenty of time.

The landlords of my nursing friend owned a couple of other rental units. We made arrangements to go look and early the next day I was on the road with one of them driving three miles back down I-5 to Dunsmuir to look at an apartment. In my opinion, Mt. Shasta appeared to be this new age, hip town with coffee, ski, and crystal shops. There was a bustle about town with people walking up and down the sidewalks and in and out of shops. Arriving in downtown Dunsmuir was just the opposite of Mt. Shasta. Dunsmuir was an old mill town that had not yet seen the up-tick in growth. The main street through town was quiet, some of the store's doors were boarded up, and it just didn't look like it would come close to meeting the needs of my dream I had been working on over the past few weeks. The apartment that I looked at was nice enough. It was a two-bedroom, one bath on the second floor of a 1940's 4-plex just off the main street, for only $250 per month. I stored that one away in my back pocket in the event I couldn't find anyplace else to live.

Later that day I stopped by the hospital to visit the pharmacy and let the director know I had made it to town and confirm my start date. While I was there, I was discussing potential living arrangements. He gave a quick phone call to his friend who just happened to be one of the administrators at the hospital. This administrator had a friend who was a teacher/builder in town who had recently built a rental property in a nice section of town. One phone call led to another and early that evening I was meeting with this guy and his wife, and they were offering to rent me this gorgeous two bedroom home in Mt. Shasta, for $375 per month. Like I said, I knew it would work out.

Papers signed and money paid, I pulled my Scout up the road from where I was staying and proceeded to back the trailer into the driveway. What an incredibly glorious feeling. My own actual house, about half a mile from downtown Mt. Shasta and less than two miles from my new job. Importantly, I was less than 15 miles away from Mt. Shasta Ski Park.

So, I took a couple days getting settled in, some used furniture, introducing myself to the neighbors and riding my mountain bike all over town. Realizing I still had four or five days before I needed to start work, I decided to go on a road trip over to the coast to visit my sister Becky and her partner Bill. With as much excitement as I can imagine, I pile a weekend worth of stuff in the convertible Scout and head down I-5 toward Redding. Next, I turn right onto 299 and head the 3-hour drive over the windy road to the coastal town of Arcata where Becky and Bill live. Well, actually they live on an amazing little ranch in the town of Fieldbrook about seven miles up into the Arcata mountains.

I am certain the trip was great, every time I visit Becky at her home is a wonderful time. Even though it was still the end of summer, I believe school had already started at Humboldt State University. Friday night was upon us, and it feels like there was a sense of football in the air. I think Humboldt was playing a game the following Saturday and the square in downtown Arcata was off-the-hook. Over the past 30 years I have been in the square maybe five or six times; however, it was never like this. College students were everywhere. It seemed like there were bars lined up all around the square, but it was the Varsity Club that Bill and Becky took me into. By the looks of the crowd that was running in and out of the bars and the way the beer was flowing, I really don't think this was a normal Friday evening for Bill and Becky, credit to them though for showing me how exciting and raucous Arcata can be on a football weekend.

By the time Sunday rolled around it was time to head back home to Mt. Shasta. Bill had graciously given me a home-built wooden desk so I would have someplace at home to put my mail and begin my writing career. We decided to head to the river in Willow Creek for a swim before I left for home. About a 45-minute drive from Bill and Becky's ranch; however, it was in the right direction toward home, so it sounded like a great idea. The river was lovely, with a slight flow so we could sit in the water and float downstream, get out, run back up and do it again.

Across the river was a cliff to climb up and I noticed a few daring folks climbing and diving off into the river. I have always been one to keep my eye open for an opportunity to jump off the side of just about anything as long as it is a clear shot to the water.

Climbing out of the water onto the cliff was no problem at all. The trail up the hill was a little concerning, with some loose and muddy silt that looked like it might pose a slipping challenge as I was about to muster my way up to the highest point. As I was working my way up, I began to slip a little, so I snagged onto this little branch poking out of the ground. As I was letting go of the twig it dawned on me that it might be a poison oak twig that had lost its leaves. No big deal, I was certain I could only get the allergic reaction from the leaves. The dive went great, and I worked my way back up the hill a couple more times before it was time to go. Hugs to Becky and Bill and I was on my way back to my awesome home in Mt. Shasta.

The following morning, I woke up in the lovely summer sunshine, warm mountain air, smell of whatever it is that grows around where I was living, and a rash. My nightmare had come true. Poison oak had started showing itself on my forearm, legs, abdomen, neck, and face. Here I am, at the beginning of a poison oak outbreak, and I need to start my first day at work tomorrow morning. Feeling absolutely mortified, I show up to work the next morning ready for orientation, with calamine lotion covering the majority of my unexposed and portions of my exposed body.

My new boss was very good natured about the entire situation. Thinking back on it, I believe he was just pleased that I had shown up and not called in sick the first day on the job. After a short discussion, he handed me a vial of dexamethasone and sent me over to the emergency room for an injection. As it was in a small community hospital in the late 80's, I walked into the emergency room, introduced myself as the new pharmacist in the hospital, and the nurse drew up the medication and gave me a deep intramuscular steroid shot. The doctor then wrote me a prescription for a tapering dose of prednisone to be taken over the next

44

eight days or so, introduced me to the emergency room staff, and sent me back to the pharmacy.

8

One Quarter Century

Two months into life in Mt. Shasta and I am about to have my 25th birthday. Nearly 60 today, 25 doesn't seem very old; however, we all know that when we are turning 25 the world is ours.

As a recognition of my time on this planet I wanted to go off and create a day long adventure worthy of 25 years. My plan was to drive up to Castle Lake, start hiking, and see where it took me. Castle lake is a glorious mountain lake about seven miles up a steep road just outside of Mt. Shasta. The air was crisp and incredibly fresh, without a cloud in the sky. The drive up to Castle Lake allows for a bit of the fall season, with quite a bit of colored foliage blowing off the trees onto the road. The views, colors, smells and temperature were all readily accessible from the cockpit of my convertible truck. As a matter of fact, I believe it was this trip that reminded me I needed to get the top bolted back onto the truck before the next rain came.

Once I reached the lake, I gathered my little pack with just a couple snacks and a bottle of water and started heading around the lake. Castle lake is about one mile long and about a half a mile wide. Not a big lake; however, it is surrounded on three sides by mountains. As you drive up to the lake you see a few semi-beach access points to the water. Looking across the lake the rock mountain juts out of the back and straight up about 1000 feet to a sloping mountain and meadows. On the right side is a sloping hill that gets increasingly steeper as it gets closer to the back of the lake.

My plan, as I was there looking at the lake, was to head left around the lake on the trail, make my way off the trail up the rocks and reach the top far to the left above the rock mountain wall. At that point, I would hike around the ridge and down the right side of the lake back to the truck. Of course, this was back when I was 25 and I didn't even think of letting anyone know where I was or what my plans were for the day.

The trail started off great, winding up and down around the lake and then made a sharp turn heading up the hill away from the lake. At that point, I looked forward toward the rocky wall and decided I wanted to continue off the trail on my own path. After a bit of creating my own way along the side of the lake I came to a boulder wall that appeared to go up maybe 500 feet toward the sloping mountain. The boulders were big, not moving, and all appeared relatively evenly spaced so they would be easy to climb from one to another. This seemed like a great way to celebrate my birthday; I had decided it would be a good idea to climb up these boulders to get to the top of the lake's ridge.

Climbing from one to another was without issue. This was simple, just get up to one boulder, look around, and find your path up to the next. After 15 or 20 minutes of this I am a little over halfway up the wall of boulders and I stop to look behind me. HOLY CRAP! Here I am, realizing that one little slip and I'll be tumbling 300 feet to a rocky demise, with only my parked Scout as an indication that I may be somewhere up here hiking on the mountain. My knees feel a bit weak and tremulous. It is very clear to me that I cannot climb back down, the only option I have is to keep climbing. With a little bit of discerning self-talk, I start my climb, and as easy as the first 100 feet I continue my climb up to the top of the boulder mountain.

As is common when hiking alone in the mountains, distances that appear short at first soon turn out to be much further than once thought. I had made it to the top of the ridge, and the views were amazing. Across the valley is Mt. Shasta. Standing tall at just over 14 thousand feet, it is covered in snow. The white volcano shaped mountain is striking against the crystal clear deep blue sky. This momentary visual distraction was lost when I realized I was still only one quarter of the way around the lake and the only way back was to continue on up the mountain slope to the top of the ridge, follow the ridge around the top of the rock wall on the far end of the lake, and then down the slope on the other side. The rest of the hike took most of the day and I was exhausted by the time I made it back to the truck. Yes, this was definitely a momentous adventure to celebrate my 25th year.

***

Living in the mountains brought with it the regular change of seasons. In Santa Cruz, we're not too familiar with season changes, being that all year we are either in spring or fall, with maybe just a little warm summer and a short cool winter. Mt. Shasta most definitely has four distinct seasons. Beginning in November I could feel the chill coming with cold mornings and dark chilly evenings. I remember that snow had come early that year with 6-12 inches out my front door sometime during the beginning of November.

Or course, being November, the snow didn't stay long and may have been melted a little by the afternoon sunshine or maybe some rain, but further up the hill it was sticking and staying. During my first few months in town, I spent quite a bit of town on my mountain bike exploring the streets as well as the fire trails that seemed to go on endlessly up, on and around the mountain. In particular, up at the end of my road, where it dead ended into the railroad tracks, a dirt road continued on the other side of the tracks.

There were many turns this way and that; however, I figured out that if I continued on the main dirt road for about five miles, I would come out on the road just below Mt. Shasta Ski Park. One Sunday morning in early November, after coffee and oatmeal, I got on my bike and started the climb up the dirt road. The air temperature was quite cold, and a light snowfall was coming down. Of course, I was dressed in my winter gear, ready for the cold and the wet. After only 10 minutes or so I was peddling in a couple inches of snow and the effort felt double what it usually did.

The beauty was a bit overwhelming. Riding my bike, a couple miles up this old fire road, snow coming down, trees and meadows blanketed in fresh snow and what seemed to be utter silence. I notice up in front of me, perhaps 100 feet or so, this enormous husky dog. There is no one else up here and the dog looks a bit mangy to be anyone's pet, and it's just standing there, still, and silent, staring at me. I'm not saying it was a wolf; well, maybe I am saying it was a wolf, not sure; however, it sure looked like a wolf to me.

It wasn't my idea to stick around and try to be friendly to it. Quickly as possible I turned my bike around and rode back to my house. Over the following few months, I told that story to some locals. They all initially laughed and said that I must have seen someone's lost dog or maybe a fox, but then they would think their way through it and maybe kind of agree with me.

***

Continuing on with the story of my first season in Mt. Shasta, at some time during the fall I had a visit from Susie and her good friend Ginger. This was fantastic! Susie and Ginger were on a personal road trip to Canada. They had the path mapped out, sleeping bags in the back of Ginger's truck, and loads of excitement. My good fortune allowed my house to be the first stop on their adventure.

I've always been so impressed that these two young ladies, both in their early 20's, packed up in a truck and headed out on a weeklong adventure, not really knowing what they would find. Stopping at grocery stores for meals and camping out of the back of a pickup truck, such a fresh way to learn about a new area.

Interestingly, they came at the same time that my brother John happened to be traveling through the area with his hang glider strapped to the top of his truck. John had some particular area he was going to launch off of and then fly across the open space, so Susie and Ginger volunteered to be his driver, meet him at the landing space and bring him back to his truck. This worked out because I think I had to work that day and it was a nice way for Susie and Ginger to see the views of the Mt. Shasta landscape.

That night we all went out for a solid Mexican meal at Lalo's, one of our local favorite restaurants. Those short two nights help solidify the relationship between Susie and me. It was my impression that she really enjoyed herself here in Mt. Shasta and liked the area. In addition, I had an actual home that was very comfortable for living. When we said goodbye and she continued on her adventure with Ginger, I felt confident we would be seeing each other again soon.

It wasn't too long after that that Susie came by herself to Mt. Shasta for a visit. She was able to stay for a few days and this gave us time to really catch up with each other, communicate, and discuss what it would be like living together. During our visit we took a trip up to Ashland, Oregon to have an exploration and see what it was like. We had a fantastic time and Susie had seen a couple of antique shops she wanted to go back and see.

Unfortunately, I had to go back to work the next day, so Susie had some time on her hands and decided to drive back up to Ashland on her own and have a look around. Somewhere on the freeway, I think it was as she was descending into Ashland, her Mustang had engine trouble and she had to pull over on the side of the freeway. UGGHHH!!! This was before cell phones, so all you could do was wait for someone to pull over and offer to help.

Again, I don't exactly remember how it all played out, but over the next couple hours Susie had her car towed down to a shop in Ashland and got herself booked into a hotel. What an amazing strong woman! She handled it. She called me at work and let me know what was going on and where she was staying. I said I would leave as soon as I got off work and drive up and stay with her for the night. She was on the phone with her step-dad Syd, who helped walk her through the steps of dealing with the shop. They had to order some parts and wouldn't have the car ready till the following afternoon.

Up early the next morning, I was on the road to get back to work at Mt. Shasta. Susie spent the day walking and exploring Ashland until her car was ready to roll. After another day or two in Mt. Shasta, she needed to get back to work herself in Santa Cruz. Again, we both knew it wasn't goodbye.

***

This takes me back specifically to my first year living in Mt. Shasta. Yes, I had skied quite a bit in high school, doing long drives to the mountains for a day of skiing accompanied with long drives back home at night. Yes, I had lived in Tahoe for the winter of 81-82 when the snow was so deep my Honda Civic looked like no more than just a bump of snow in the driveway. Mt. Shasta, during that first year, was different. This was my time to ski.

Snow came early in the winter of 88-89 in Northern California. By the third week of January over two feet of snow had accumulated in downtown Mt. Shasta and Mt. Shasta Ski Park was opening the weekend before Thanksgiving. Unlike my year in Tahoe, this time I had a 4-wheel drive to get up to the mountain, a full access season pass and a brand-new pair of skis and boots. Every free day I had was spent up on the mountain skiing. As well, the ski park had a Wednesday evening race series that I joined and participated in on a weekly basis.

Throughout the year I made quite a few acquaintances who skied regularly. On any given day I would find a friend in the lift line, and we would do some runs together. Following all of these different individuals down the mountain helped me gain my skiing ability. These are the days where I truly developed my muscle memory that I am able to call upon these days in order to remember how to float through powder or slide down between bumps after being off my skis for over a year.

***

After being in Mt. Shasta for maybe only a month or so I met a dear soul of a man who worked as a nurse at the hospital. Jim Patterson was 11 years my senior; however, we had some sort of intrinsic connection that allowed us the opportunity to create long, interesting, and meaningful conversations. Jim was recently separated in a relationship and lived less than a mile from my house, so this was a good time in life for both of us to hang out together.

In Jim's garage he had a ping pong table. My skills were relatively stable; however, Jim had a hand-paddle-ball coordination that was fantastic. We created an abacus of string and washers that hung across the garage to keep track of our game count and would regularly play well into the night with beer and music, regularly stopping to debate interesting topics that would arise.

Over the six years that Susie and I lived in Mt. Shasta Jim was an integral part of our life. After leaving Mt. Shasta we got together two times, once in Santa Cruz and once in Mt. Shasta. Unfortunately, we were neglectful in keeping in touch and Jim passed away from a sudden heart attack in 2016. He will always hold a special place in both mine and Susie's heart.

9

Susie

By nature, I am a social person. Throughout the fall and winter of 88/89, I had made friends and was developing a social circle. It became clear to me that I really missed Susie and I wanted her to move up to Mt. Shasta and create a life with me. It's hard to put into words how much I admired Susie. She had created this life of hers, all on her own, and seemed to do just fine without me. This only made me want her more.

April 1st, 1989, Susie packed her car and moved to Mt. Shasta to move in with me. More than moving out on my own, more than living in Boston for six months, more than having keys to a pharmacy at 23 years old, Susie moving in with me was by far the biggest thing that had ever happened in my life. Deep inside I knew I loved Susie and somehow knew I would spend the rest of my life with her. On the other hand, I still had my hot wheel race cars, mountain bike and skis as decoration in the living room. I had a lot to learn.

Susie brought with her a freshness that was so desperately needed. Before I knew it, we had plants in the house and the dining room table was decorated. The bathroom counter had all sorts of new items on it, and I found it was now necessary to separate clothes into certain categories before putting them in the washing machine.

It didn't take long at all, and Susie had a job working for a local hot tub sales office. Of course, even though she was great at her work, a few months later she settled into a job with a local medical clinic where she was able to use her skills from all the years working at the Scotts Valley Medical Clinic.

Our first spring together in Mt. Shasta was nothing short of a continuous adventure. Of course, the ski season wasn't over yet, so we had a couple of wonderful days skiing at the Mt. Shasta ski park. Much to her credit, Susie had developed some good skills from her days in Tahoe.

As an aside note; when Susie was young her parents went in halves on a cabin in South Lake Tahoe along with another couple. She tells stories of her mom and Dad taking them down to the lake, riding bikes, and having fun summers and winters in Tahoe. Later, as she got into high school, she would head up to the cabin with her friends during winter and go skiing. Funny thing is, my mom and Dad rented the cabin from them when I was in junior high and high school. We went up a couple times during the summer as well as winter. It wasn't until after we were living together in Mt. Shasta that we put two and two together to figure this out.

Every weekend we would plan some type of hike or drive around the local area; exploring the road up the mountain to the old ski park, hiking the Eddy's and the Dead Fall lakes, Castle Crags, jumping in the water at the McCloud River Falls, and exploring the towns of Yreka, Weed, Dunsmuir, and Redding. The most fun; however, was one of our regular after work or weekend jaunts down to the shores of lake Siskiyou. Just one or two miles out of town, the lake has multiple spots where we could park and just walk a short distance down to a sandy or rocky beach on the beautiful shoreline.

During the warm spring days or the sizzling hot summer heat waves, trips to the lake were met with excited anticipation. About 5pm, after we have both come home from work, maybe early June, the sun is still high in the sky and the temperature is in the mid 80's. Susie is wearing her shorts, sneakers, and a bikini top and I have my swimsuit and sneakers on. We are in the Scout, top off, driving through downtown Mt. Shasta heading out to the lake.

We find our spot to pull off the road, a little turn out in the shade about 100 yards up from the lake. We step over a little cable hung between two poles and stroll, hand in hand, down the shaded trail through the trees to the lake. As per usual, Susie sets her towel down and takes a seat while I toss my towel on the sand and go straight into the water. Of course, after a few minutes Susie quickly joins me, cooling herself off from the heat in the lovely water.

Susie and I have spent lots of time together over the years. We still walk hand in hand wherever we go. Neither of us are particularly chatty; however, we spend hours and hours talking with each other. We are both rather sensitive and neither of us ever means to hurt the other; however, it happens. Many times, over the years we have had multiple hour-long talks, peeling away layers of emotions, filled with tears, diving deep into each other's reason for being and staying in this relationship. Each and every time it comes back to how we make each other feel.

Like just about everyone else in the world, both Susie and I have deep seated emotions from past life experiences. These emotions and experiences have a strong influence, whether we know it or not, over how we act in current and future relationships. As we age, God willing, we will have had opportunities to examine these emotions and experiences and be in a better position to use them positively when we communicate with those we love. When we are younger, like in our mid 20's as Susie and I were when we moved in with each other, we may not be as in touch with our emotional influences as we think we are.

What I'm trying to say is that during those early years our deep communication was a little rough. Through my teens and college, I worked at becoming a better listener and communicator; however, I think I took it as more of a competition rather than a two-way communication street. Susie brought a new angle to all of this. She had this deep level of understanding and was ready to share back and forth, and assumed I knew that this was a thing and knew how to do this. This took many years to unfold and I'm getting ahead of myself a little here. Through many hours, days, weeks, months, and years of going back and forth with each other, through laughter, pain, and tears, we have grown to a place I feel not many couples experience. We have grown into a relationship that I always wanted but never knew existed. I'll get back to this emotional pull between Susie and I later in the book, but for now, I need to get back into the timeline before I'm lost in the ever-evolving relationship with my dear wife.

***

By the summer of 89' Susie and I had been living with each other for well over four months. Yes, I know four months isn't long; however, we were 26 and 25 years old at the time and a few months nearly constitutes a lifetime at that point in life. As happens, we found ourselves looking to create a home of our own. One afternoon Susie was out and found a cute old farmhouse just about a mile past the hospital on the way out of town. An old school farmhouse with this rustic wrap around porch looking out over the lilacs and circle driveway.

After not much discussion we decided this was the home for us. We contacted a real estate agent and looked at the home situated on a flat acre of property with views of Mt. Shasta and started planning on how we could make an offer. The price was $59,000, which at the time in 1989, seemed like a reasonable deal. The issue was, Susie and I could only come up with half of the 20% down payment. Interestingly, as if it were meant to happen, our real estate agent stepped in. She and her husband had just moved into the area, and she really wanted to make her first sale. In addition, she said she had this sense about people, and she really liked us. Our offer to purchase the house was accepted with the real estate agent loaning us the other 50% of the down payment on a 12 month note.

Susie and I were now homeowners. It's hard to put into words how we felt. This was incredibly exciting for us, creating our own home together. Honestly though, we had little to zero idea of what we were getting ourselves into. This home, built in the mid 30's, had no insulation, single pane windows, support posts sitting on dirt in many places, and the only heat was a wood stove. That first winter was either frigid cold from no

56

fire, or the doors and windows were open because we had a roaring fire that heated up the entire neighborhood. We must have gone through six or seven cords of wood that first winter.

Not to bore you with all the specifics, but over the first two years we both learned more than we ever thought we would about hiring work done on a home and doing work for ourselves. New foundation, storm windows all around, insulation under the house, in the ceiling, and blown into the walls, new heater and fireplace, never ending cosmetic renovation; just a constant process of creating our new home.

One day in the fall, while I was at work, I happened to be in the emergency room when someone brought in a black Labrador puppy. For some horrible reason, this puppy had been left on the side of the freeway. Fortunately, someone saw him, stopped, and picked him up, then brought him to the hospital. The moment I heard the story I was on the phone to Susie asking her if she would like to have a dog. Of course, she said yes. She happened to be off of work that day and came down to the hospital to pick him up. After just a short bit of discussion, we came up with the name Rolf. Since that time, dogs have been a constant part of our life and sitting at my feet, Nico and Lucy are our 9th and 10th canine editions to our home.

During those early years Susie and I were quite ambitious. We were both new at this home making business and we weren't sure there were any specific rules to how we could do it. For example, we painted our bathroom lime green with stripes on one wall. As well, we cut a hole in our living room ceiling and framed a bridge upstairs to go from the front half of our bedroom to the back half of our bedroom. As a pharmacist, I had zero prior knowledge on how to build and frame; however, I knew how to read books and with Susie as my partner, we figured it out. We cut the hole, framed it in, put in some support and made it our own.

One of our favorite homes making adventures was actually a landscape endeavor. About three miles down the road, around Lake Siskiyou and up the creek a little way we found an excellent supply of river rock. We would take the Scout and follow a little dirt road off the main (not so main) road, and it wound its way down to an immense rocky section of river. Next, we would begin the process of gathering these 20- and 30-pound river rocks to load in the back of the Scout. One trip, start to finish, would probably take two or three hours; however, it was great hang out time and we really enjoyed the beautiful surroundings. When we got back to our home, we would commence lining the driveway with these rocks. Really, it looked gorgeous.

As I was discussing earlier, our communication in our younger years was a bit rough. Well, I believe it was my ability to communicate my emotions and needs that was a bit rough. Susie, given the opportunity, was willing to listen and communicate her emotions; however, perhaps sometimes I overrode them a bit.

It was after one of these long river rock adventure trips that I somehow, I got the picture that I needed to either move forward with the relationship with a deeper commitment or let her go. I knew right then and there that this was our life, whether it was collecting river rock, rescuing Labradors, renovating homes or any of the other future adventures I had no knowledge of. Without much planning, on 10/10/1989 I got down on my knee and proposed to Susie. Without any hesitation she said YES!

Honestly, I can say that some of the most exciting times in a couple's life is the time between when they become engaged and the time when they become married. This incredible feeling that we are beginning an adult life with plans of building a home and creating a family. Of course, there are many steps, plans and discussions between the two points.

After quite a bit of communication we decided we would like to be married in the Catholic church. We talked with Father Miles, or local priest at St. Anthony's church in Mt. Shasta. Of course, he was very excited for us; however, he did lay out the steps we needed to go through. For his part, I could tell that he felt it just a bit un-orthodox that we had already moved in together before we had started this marriage path; however, to his credit, he didn't dwell on the subject and quickly got on with the business at hand.

The first step was that Susie needed to continue through the sacrament of confirmation. She went to her classes, met with the priest as necessary, and then went through a confirmation ceremony at church; absolutely beautiful. Next, Susie and I attended a series of marriage classes with Father Miles. We would go over to his house every week in the evening and talk through whichever subject he had at the time. This was a great process, but like all things educational, quite often the class work is filed away in the back of the closet and when you need it you might not remember where you put it.

We had this idea that we would like to be married outside. Our yard at our house was beautiful and had more than enough space. We proposed the idea to Father Miles. He was not against it; however, he stated we would need to first get the approval of the bishop down in Sacramento. Being a little naive, I wrote the bishop a letter explaining what we would like to do. Very eloquently the bishop described that, although he appreciated our desire, if he let the cat out of the bag it would be out forever. Long story short, he stated that if we wanted to be married by the Catholic church, we needed to be married inside a Catholic church. This was fine with us. We continued with our plan to be married on July 7th, 1990, in St. Anthony's church. We decided we would incorporate our yard by having our wedding reception at our house outside in our 1-acre garden-park-yard.

Let's see if I can do our wedding justice in my writing. Sitting here thinking about it I am not sure I can. I have started this paragraph over and over and deleted the words. By no means was our wedding limited in fashion at all. First, we had a full mass, and the wedding went on for over 90 minutes; kneeling, standing, all the prayers, communion, the works. Susie and I each had a full complement of bride's maids and grooms' men filling up the entire church altar. The church was packed, standing room only, with just about every family member (brothers, sisters, aunts, uncles, nephews, nieces, parents, and grandparents) we knew from both sides of our family. As well, we had all our new friends from Mt. Shasta and dozens of friends who had come in from out of town for the weekend. For music we had this great string quartet of musicians that Susie worked with who played amazing music filled with love. We also had my brother and his wife sing Crystal Blue Persuasion which sounded like angels flying through the church.

As I am standing in the vestibule, waiting for the groom and his men to walk down the aisle, when Father Miles asks me for the marriage certificate. I looked at him, felt my back pocket, then realized I had left it at home. I looked at Father Miles as if to ask him if it could wait and before I could even ask him, he was telling me I needed to go get it. Without hesitation I ran out of the front of the church, jumped into the convertible Scout, and raced off down the road toward home to get our marriage license. Later I find out that Susie was watching from across the street in the rectory, halfway wondering if I was making a break for it!

We're back at the church, standing down at the altar with my best man, Danny, and grooms' men, Dana, Jim, Dave, and David, and I hear the music change from casual entertainment to the wedding march. I see Susie, with her stepfather Syd on one side and Gramps on the other, walking down the aisle toward me. Such an amazingly beautiful lady. Even now, just thinking and remembering about it, I begin to get choked up. As Susie will attest to, I have a way of getting choked up over the simplest of things, and this was explicitly more than the simplest of things.

The wedding ceremony went beautifully. Even the moment when the ring bearer, Kyle, brought the ring up on the pillow and the knot was tied so tight I couldn't get the ring off. One of Susie's cousins stepped up with his buck knife and quickly cut the ribbon from the pillow releasing the wedding ring for me. My memory of our wedding is all the most wonderful things in the world packed into one experience. The ceremony of mass, the ceremony of the wedding, the candles, readings, songs, prayers, people, pictures after; just all of it.

By midafternoon we had all returned to our house for the wedding party. Dee, Susie's Mom, had single handedly masterminded the food production. We were both so incredibly grateful for the magnificent spread of food she had orchestrated and put together. Well over 150 people in our backyard and more food than everyone could finish.

Our yard had been beautifully manicured over the past few weeks. I had spent hours mowing the lawn and cleaning the yard, with anticipation of an event no one would soon forget. Banquet tables had been spread across the back side of the house with room enough for everyone to have a place to sit. The volleyball court was in full play and as I think back, the entire yard was full of happy friends and family, spread across the tables and lawn, enjoying the sunshine, drinking, eating, and celebrating our wedding.

We had hired a couple of guys to come up from Redding to run the music for us. Early evening, we got the grassy dance floor moving with sets of music from the 80's. Before long it felt like everyone at the reception was moving and grooving to the tunes. Susie and I had our official wedding dance to the smooth sound of Crystal Blue Persuasion, which was soon followed by our unofficial wedding dance to the rocking' AC/DC song, You Shook Me All Night Long. During the latter, Susie and I took over the entire dance floor with our high energy dancing.

During the afternoon and evening Susie and I did our best to walk through and take time with each and every group of people that had shown up. Mt. Shasta isn't just around the corner, friends and family needed to drive hundreds of miles to the northern tip of California for this wedding. This was an incredibly special feeling for both of us, that our family would go to such great lengths to participate in our marriage ceremony. We wanted to do our best to show them all how much we appreciated and respected their efforts at making it to our celebration day. As a matter of fact, we showed so much appreciation that by 10pm they all had to kick us out of the party so they could all go back to their hotels and get some rest. Susie and I were having such a great time that we didn't realize how late it had become. We had quite a few friends who needed places to stay so some camped in our back yard while others took over our house for the night. Susie's stepbrother, Brian, put us in his car and drove us off to the little motel room we had rented for our honeymoon night.

We hadn't done much planning for the next morning. After we finally awoke and got going mid-morning, Susie and I put on our shorts, t-shirts, and shoes, packed our wedding clothes in our backpack and hiked about a half mile through town back to my mom and Dad's house. I guess now is a good time to bring up that my mom and Dad just happened to move to Mt. Shasta only a few months after Susie moved in with me. This scenario needs a bit of explaining and will need to wait for the next chapter.

Susie and I are now married, we have a magnificent brunch at our home, with all our friends and family who have stayed over. After we have cleaned up and packed, we are soon on the road in Susie's mustang headed for San Francisco to begin our honeymoon. That night we stayed at a little hotel near the San Francisco airport and early the next morning we are on our way to Kauai for an amazing 2-week vacation.

At 26 years old I felt like I was well on my way to accomplishing life's goals; professional license and job that I felt passionate about, purchase of a home, and marriage with the love of my life. Unfortunately, much to my discern and consternation, I had yet to even get a glimpse of what my fears looked like or how they would manifest and alter our life over the next seven years.

Fears, yes, those nasty feelings that manifest because we are far too deeply concerned about what others think of us and, if masked rather than faced, quite often lead to dishonest behavior. This may sound a little dark, well, because it is however, not to fear, there is a bright light at the end of the tunnel. Before we talk about this; however, first we must remember what it was like having Mom and Dad move in down the street from us as well as the birth of our two beautiful and loving children.

10

Cooper and Kendyl

Both Susie and I know the night each of our children were conceived. I'm not sure this is normal with parents, maybe it is; however, it is clear to us. That said, it is not my intention to go into the story behind each of these, just know that we know. Now, as a parent looking back, it really doesn't seem that long ago; however, if I go back and put myself in the time when they were born, I get an entirely different perspective on the time frame.

On the 4th of July 1991, three days before our 1-year anniversary, Susie and I walked in the Mt. Shasta 5K town race. What an exciting event. The sun was shining bright, warm weather, and the young 28-year-old Steven and 27-year-old Susie were holding hands enjoying the walk. Noticeably, Susie was eight months pregnant. Just a little more than a month later, right after I had come home from work, we went out for a little walk. Not very far into the walk Susie let me know that it was time to get to the hospital, we had a baby on the way.

By the time Susie got settled into the hospital bed and started contractions it was maybe about 10 or 10: 30 pm. Things progressed quickly from that point. Just after midnight, on 8/7/1991, Susie was well into the contractions, doing her best to remember the breathing techniques we had practiced at birthing class just a few weeks prior. By this time, we had Susie's good friend Cindy in the room for support, as well as our good friend Jim who participated by filming the entire event on a VHS recorder.

Certainly, I would not say it was easy, I wasn't the one giving birth, and by the looks of things, it's never easy. I can say that the birth was without incident and happened relatively quickly in the whole scheme of things. It wasn't long and Kendyl Marie Leuck was resting on her mother. What an incredibly beautiful sight.

Less than 24 hours in the hospital and we were home with a baby, just like that. This was truly a magical time in our life. Susie and I adored our new baby and wanted her to experience life with us. Thinking back, it doesn't feel like having a little newborn girl with us slowed us down much. We still went to the lake to go swimming, we took her with us out to dinner, we went for hikes, and we even went cross country skiing across a frozen lake with our 1-year-old in a backpack.

Early in the fall, when Kendyl was maybe two or three months old, Susie went to Redding for the day with a couple friends. I have an amazing memory of resting with Kendyl on the hammock on the front porch of our Lassen Lane home. We were in the shade; however, it was still warm. I remember the amazing feeling of having a baby sleeping on you and how we do all we possibly can to protect them.

About one year after Kendyl was born, and only three years since we had moved into our lovely farmhouse, we moved. I was restless. We were living in an old farmhouse; however, it could have been updated and made into a nice warm home. I felt like we would do better to move into a nice new home that was all completed and ready for us to raise our family in. Our current house was high maintenance, so Susie and I started looking at some of the new homes in the area. We walked into this lovely home and were immediately infatuated with the house. It was hard to believe that people actually lived in houses this nice, and that we would soon be living here.

Before long we had left the simple life of living in a farmhouse and were now settling into an upscale custom home with windows looking out over all the beautiful mountains. Susie was now pregnant with our second child; we had room to grow in our new home. Kendyl's bedroom had just about tripled in size from her bedroom on Lassen Lane.

Here's the other side of the story. I had recently taken a management position in the pharmacy at the hospital. At 28 years old, I was younger than the two pharmacists and four technicians I was managing. My training to become a manager was negligible, and furthermore, my stealth drug use was in a growth spurt. All of this added to the fact that I was becoming increasingly unavailable to my wife for both emotional and physical support. My ability to provide financial support for my family led me to believe, falsely, that I was available to them as a supporting and understanding husband and father.

During the nine months pregnant with Cooper, I can only imagine that Susie must have felt like she was increasingly needing to do this on her own. As I managed the pharmacy, worked long hours, and brought work home, Susie managed the house and Kendyl.

Yes, we did had loving and happy moments during this time; however, life was difficult. Kendyl was developing her lovely personality and wanted to stay up late. I was not taking care of my physical body and was tired. Regularly, Susie would get up out of bed, pregnant, and go sit with Kendyl so I could sleep and be ready for work the next day. This was far from fair. Susie had worked hard, if not harder, all day long and now she is covering for me at nighttime as well.

Cooper Steven Leuck came faster than Kendyl. When we got to the hospital, we didn't have time to call Jim with the VHS recorder, it was all business. The cool thing is Susie's doctor had me deliver Cooper. He was sitting right behind me with his hands basically over the top of my hands; however, I caught Cooper's head as it came out, helped his first shoulder, then the next and pulled his body up and out and laid him down on top of Susie's front side. Absolutely one of the most amazing moments in our life.

We brought Cooper home to our big fancy house and proceeded to do the best we could at raising our two children. I am eternally grateful for the effort Susie put forward that year, keeping the house and family together. As well, we were incredibly fortunate to have Mom and Dad just a mile away for support. Of course, during this time Mom was medically challenged and was taking most of Dad's time and attention; however, nothing brightened their day more than Susie bringing Cooper and Kendyl over for an afternoon visit.

11

Larry and Dorie

Mom and Dad moved from their life in Southern California to Ben Lomond during the summer of 1962. With seven children, ages 5-17, they created a home in a rental house in the Ben Lomond mountains. Dad had a job over the hill in Sunnyvale, which took him more than an hour to get to; however, he and Mom were positive this move was right for the family.

The winters were long, dark, and wet in the 60's in the Santa Cruz mountains, especially living at the top of the road on the outskirts of Ben Lomond. One of these dark evenings in February of 1963, with a house full of seven kids roaming around the house, Mom in her early 40's and Dad in his late 40's, with rain pouring so hard that you wouldn't believe it unless you had grown up in Ben Lomond, Mom looked at Dad and said, Larry, I'm pregnant.

By the end of summer Mom and Dad had purchased the big house in downtown Ben Lomond, right on the river and next to the castle. Then, October 20th, 1963, little Steven was born. For the next 25 years this house was home for Larry and Dorie.

With all of their eight children graduated high school and moving on with their lives, it was now time for Mom and Dad to sell the big home and start the next chapter of their life.

Sometime during 1988 Mom and Dad sold their home, put most of their belongings in storage, and moved to South Lake Tahoe to live in Lydia and Harry's vacation home. To their good fortune, their timing was great, for had they waited much longer they would have been significantly affected by the Loma Prieto earthquake of 1989 that shook Santa Cruz like a rag doll.

Mom and Dad enjoyed Tahoe; however, they wanted to be near some family. Sometime around the summer of 1989 they decided they would do a tour throughout California and visit their children while also having a look around the local area to see if it might be a suitable location for an extended retirement. Mt. Shasta being in the north part of the state and not an unrealistic drive from South Lake Tahoe, they decided their visit with us would be the first stop on their tour.

Earlier in the year they had come to visit for a few days, so they already had an idea of the town. Perhaps they had some conversations between themselves about the local area already and had come to some sort of decision, I'll never know. What I do know is they came for another visit, looked around town for maybe two days, met with a real-estate agent, and bought a house. This house met all of Mom's specific requirements. The house was right next door to St. Anthony's Catholic Church, walking distance to the grocery store, and less than two blocks from the hospital.

It didn't take them very long and they had remodeled the upstairs, had all their belongings shipped from storage, and made it their home. Mt. Shasta had become, overnight, the new gathering place for the Leuck family. Brothers and sisters, their spouses, and children, all began coming on a regular basis to visit Mom and Dad in their new home, and yes, Steve and Susie as well.

Thinking back, I have a hard time imagining how Susie must have felt, having my mom and Dad move into town only a few months after she moved into town to live with their youngest son. Whatever uncomfortable feeling there may have been at the beginning of this chapter of life, Susie did an amazing job of smoothing it all over and creating a loving, healthy, and happy relationship.

From the beginning, Susie made Mom and Dad feel comfortable, and Mom and Dad did the same with Susie. This was a good thing because for our six years in Mt. Shasta, we spent quite a bit of time hanging out with each other.

Growing up in Ben Lomond our front door was never locked. Families would stop by unannounced all the time, mostly at reasonable hours; however, it was not unforeseeable that a brother or sister and their partner may come over or stop by early in the morning or late at night. The door would be unlocked, and they would just walk in. This was normal. This was how we grew up.

Come to find out, this isn't normal for most people. Most people, family or not, call first or at least knock before entering the house of a family member. This took Susie a bit of time to get familiar with. Mom and Dad would stop by, just being out on a drive in the beautiful countryside, and come on in. This was not a bad thing by any stretch; however, it was a new thing for Susie. Rather than make a big deal out of it, she saw it for what it was; loving parents wanting to share a bit of their life with their son and his wonderful wife. Susie quickly learned to check and make sure the doors were locked before she jumped in the shower!

From the first day Mom and Dad moved into town they were supportive of Susie and I living together. They were incredibly loving and non-judgmental in both their words and actions. This only amplified the joy on their faces when, on October 10th, 1989, after proposing to Susie, we walked the 1-mile distance from our house to their house to tell them the fantastic news. It just so happens that October 10th is the anniversary of Mom and Dad's marriage.

Throughout the Mt. Shasta years, Susie and I got to see glimpses of what a young couple was once beginning to date again. They had moved from their Ben Lomond house of 25 years and were now, essentially, on their own again without kids. They would take drives to the nearby towns to go shopping or go out to lunch. It was always so nice to see how they treated each other with love and respect.

***

One of the early Halloweens Susie and I had a costume party to go to, so Mom and Dad offered to come over and watch our 10-week-old daughter. Kendyl is active, exciting, and the absolute center of attention at any gathering. Importantly, she is the only grandchild within 250 miles of Mom and Dad, so, of course you understand the attraction.

Susie was dressed as the most beautiful peacock you could ever imagine, with this tight-fitting purple body suit and peacock feathers coming up in a flume off her back side. I was dressed as a cat, in hot pursuit of the bird. Soon Mom and Dad come to the door, unexpectedly, in complete costume. We had just expected them to come over and hang out while we were gone for a couple hours; however, standing in front of us, was an exact replica of Saddam Hussein and his wife. Complete with makeup and costume from head to toe, they looked great. It was clearly obvious they had tons of fun taking the time to dress up and put the costume together.

***

Susie and I had an acre of flat property at our Lassen Lane home. After a few months, we got the idea that it would be great to water the entire property on a regular basis, so the grass would grow lush and green, and we could mow it. Obviously, we were young and hadn't thought through the long game of watering an acre of property and all the time and effort it takes to maintain a grassy park like setting, we just wanted to create a nice spot to hang out in the yard. We did it, we created a beautiful park-like setting, and it was great. Building this; however, was a bit of work.

Susie helped me plot out the property with graph paper. Next, we bought a book to learn about sprinkler systems. After a little bit of study time, we went out to the yard and plotted out over 12 different sprinkler zones and 35 separate sprinkler heads. Seemed reasonable at the time. I'm not sure how many feet of plc. pipe we had to purchase; however, it all needed to be buried at least 18 inches in the ground.

After plotting out the ground, I started digging. Before work, after work, weekends, for one entire month I dug trenches around the property. Dad would come over on a regular basis to check on my progress. He completely enjoyed seeing his youngest son work on a home. At the time I didn't really understand why; but now, I look forward to the opportunity to visit with my son when he is working on a project at his home. Dad would give some ideas, offer encouragement, and tell stories. Mostly he would talk about things that had happened in his life that came up because something we were doing reminded him of it. This was great.

It was during one of these visits, out digging in the yard, that Dad gave me one of the most important pieces of advice he ever said, "Steven, if you just keep digging, before you know it, you'll be done." So very incredibly simple yet so very true. Many times, in my life since that point, I have used that phrase to keep me going to finish a project. Whatever the project may be, if you just keep doing it, and don't give up, you'll eventually finish it.

***

During Kendyl's first three years, as well as Cooper's first year, they both had the amazing fortune of having both my Mom and Dad in their lives. Dad loved going for walks, he has always loved going for walks, as long as I can remember. From the time when I was four years old, I would catch him at the door as soon as he came home from work and would ask him to walk me to the park, through high school when we would go on after dinner walks around Old County Road or up to the post office in Ben Lomond.

Beginning with Kendyl, Dad would take her on long strolls, whether he had her in the fancy three wheeled baby jogger that could travel over dirt roads or was carrying her, he would regularly work his way up to the train tracks and walk her through town. During our last year in Mt.

Shasta, when Cooper was born, Dad didn't have quite as much time or energy. His time was mostly spent taking care of Mom as she was decreasing in her abilities to manage her daily functions. Even so, we would stop by and visit on a regular basis and the excitement and love that was shared from Mom and Dad to our children is something we will all feel deep inside us for the rest of our lives.

Susie and I can clearly remember, visiting Mom and Dad for dinner. Mom would gather Kendyl in her arms in the kitchen and plop her right down in the middle of the kitchen island. She would then proceed to scoop her finger through the butter on the counter and hold her finger up for Kendyl to lick off. I know, this sounds a little disgusting; however, it was true joy and happiness for both Kendyl and Mom.

Throughout the late spring, summer and early fall we would regularly gather as a group and head down to Lake Siskiyou for an afternoon picnic and swim. The north shore of the lake was a regular gathering spot for us, especially when family came into town. We would pull off onto the dirt road, drive around the lake about two miles through this dusty road through the trees, and come out at this amazing open meadow area the size of three football fields. We Park up above and then just walk down to wherever you find a nice spot and set up a day camp. Both Susie and Mom would create lovely snacks for all of us to eat and we had such a great time playing in the lake.

***

Sometimes I felt like God had guided me through pharmacy school so I could be present to help mom take care of her medications. Not long after they moved in I would, weekly, help Mom lay out her medications for the week. Up to this point, Mom had given birth to eight children, was diagnosed with rheumatoid arthritis and lupus, and had multiple surgeries, including multiple bowel surgeries and heart valve replacement in 1980. This is to say, she was familiar with medical clinics and hospitals, and it was no surprise the first time she was a patient in the hospital where I was a pharmacist.

It is difficult to recall the exact timeline; however, sometime during the early Mt. Shasta years Mom needed to have her heart valve replaced again. Of course, it took a few visits to the local hospital before they came to that conclusion. It just so happens that during one of these visits to the hospital, Susie was also in the hospital ready to give birth to Kendyl. How lovely it was during the early morning hours when the nurse wheeled Mom over to Susie's room to see Kendyl, less than 10 hours old.

Soon after, Mom was taken up to Medford, Oregon to a regional medical center for her heart surgery. It feels like she was there for two weeks, and Dad made the trip up and back, accompanied by one of their many children, many times. Mom and Dad did well at having many children, they always had at least one of them, or their spouse/partner, present when they needed them. Mom recovered well from surgery, came home, and continued on as she always had.

There were times when Mom would be admitted to the hospital and be taken directly to the Intensive Care Unit with the purpose of stabilizing her heart rate and fluid congestion.

Weekend coverage at this hospital, at the time, was rotated between the two staff pharmacists. We would cover the shift, with the help of two technicians, from 8am to 4:30pm and then give the charge nurse our phone number if there were any issues that came up overnight. It was not a large hospital, with only four intensive care unit (ICU) beds, 20 acute care beds and a 50-bed skilled nursing unit.

With mom being a frequent flier to the local community hospital, it was not uncommon for me to be the pharmacist on duty for the weekend while mom happened to be an inpatient in the hospital for one reason or another.

This particular weekend, Mom was in the ICU following a surgery, when I heard the announcement over the intercom system "Code Blue, ICU". At the time I was 26 years old and had attended and participated in many Codes Blue events, so I didn't think twice. I grabbed my calculator and got myself down to the ICU in a hurry.

Upon entering the unit, there was Mom, with her gown stripped off and a nurse leaning over her side administering chest compressions. The scene was like any other Code Blue event, with three nurses, the physician who just happened to be in the ICU at the time, the anesthesiologist who happened to be on his Saturday afternoon pain rounds, and the respiratory therapist called away from administering a breathing treatment.

The difference this time; this was my Mom.

The first step was to pull the emergency medication tray out of the crash cart. I was pulling the plastic off the tray in preparation of the first medication order when the anesthesiologist looked my way and said, "Should he be in here"? I was quick to reply, "I'm good", and that's all that was said.

Who else was going to do this, I thought? I am the pharmacist on duty; I am the one who knows where everything is, the dosing calculations, and how to mix the medications. The Code went on for 30 minutes or more. Mom was stabilized; however, it was not easy. After a few days she was discharged home and life, as she knew it, went back to normal.

I was young and not prepared for how this process would affect me. The moment I said, "I'm good", I unknowingly made an agreement with myself to treat my mother as a patient, as opposed to being present as a loving son.

At the time, I was unaware of the great effort I employed to suppress the immediate surging emotions. I was successful at suppressing these emotions and was able to perform appropriately during the crisis. The challenge was, these emotions were suppressed so firmly, it took years to bring them back up to the surface to be recognized and dealt with in a loving manner.

Yes, my personal situation was a little extreme; however, upon retrospection I have found that my objective behavior may have been a little skewed, to say the least. I feel confident, had I stepped out of the room, the staff would have managed the emergency medications appropriately.

Nearly 30 years ago, I can still feel the emotions as if it were yesterday. We learn lessons throughout our life. If we are fortunate, at some point we are able to take the meaning from the lesson and place it in our toolbox. When difficult situations arise, we then take a glance into that toolbox and see what lessons we have stored away that may be applied to our current situation.

***

As well, Dad had his share of encounters with the Mt. Shasta medical team, albeit a little less dramatic. One particular situation Dad was troubled with was chest pain. He had a physician named Dr. Cleaver. Yes, his name was actually Dr. Cleaver. Sounds like a character out of Young Frankenstein or some other classic monster comedy. Regardless, Dr. Cleaver did his best to take care of Dad.

One morning during one of our final winters in Mt. Shasta I stopped by Mom and Dad's house just to check in and see how they were doing. This was mid-January and the snow had fallen nearly six feet over the past few days in downtown Mt. Shasta. The snowplow had yet to drive down Dad's alley by the side of his house, so his car was stuck under the snow, and at least 15 feet to go to get it out.

There was Dad, the never-ending worker, with his shovel in hand tossing endless amounts of snow off to the side with hopes of gaining access to the main road for his blue Buick. As I was walking over to visit, and relieve him of the shovel, I noticed him take out a little bottle of pills from his pocket, open the bottle, and pop one under his tongue. Of course, I realized these were nitroglycerine pills and they are used to help relieve sharp chest pain due to narrowing of the arteries in the heart. My concern, as a pharmacist and a son, to see Dad popping a nitroglycerine pill while at the same time shoveling snow was significant. Looking at Dad, I could not recognize any concern whatsoever so I thought I would ask him about it.

Nonchalantly, so as not to raise concern, I asked Dad how often he experienced significant enough chest pain to use one of these pills. He responded, again very nonchalantly, saying about eight or nine times a day. Apparently, Dr. Cleaver and Dad had come to an understanding. Dr. Cleaver knew Dad had significant chest pain and decreased blood flow to his heart. He had told Dad to just go ahead and use the pills as often as he needed.

Dad had alluded to a conversation he had with Dr. Cleaver where the good doctor had explained to Larry that, well, he is in his late 70's and has lived a good life. I'm not certain how the conversation went after that; however, it appears that Dr. Cleaver had directed Dad into just living with his heart condition and treating the symptoms, rather than sending him to a cardiac center in either Redding or Medford to have his condition evaluated.

Within the next year, after Dad had moved back down to Santa Cruz, he was able to get into see a cardiologist for a thorough examination. Soon after the exam, he was in the cardiac care unit at Dominican Hospital undergoing cardiac bypass surgery for severe blockage. Dad went on to live about 10 more years after that surgery, all of them without any chest pain.

***

During their six years living in Mt. Shasta, we had fantastic visits, great meals together, super fun family gatherings with brothers and sisters, nephews and nieces coming to stay, and it all happened in and around Mom having a progressively worsening medical condition.

Sometime during the first three years Mom had about a 12 month long urinary tract infection. This was frustrating to her, to say the least. She would develop significant symptoms, go to the doctor, go to the lab for blood work, receive antibiotics and improve over the course of two weeks. Then, as soon as she stopped her antibiotics, the cycle would happen again.

All along she was having a decreased ability to eat due to chronic bowel pain. Her lack of eating was, initially, bringing her down to the weight she had wanted to be for such a long time; however, she passed that weight and just began getting small. I'm not certain exactly how they came to the diagnosis, but the medical team of doctors working with Mom figured out she had a large diverticulum in her small intestine that had grown to the size of a grapefruit with a hardened point. This hardened point had punctured her bladder and was slowly and constantly dripping bowel contents into her urinary tract.

Mom had to undergo an exploratory bowel surgery in order to remove the diverticula and patch up the bowel. Unfortunately, the damage to her intestinal tract was significant and the bowel needed to be redirected, out of the body into an ostomy bag. To just about anyone else, this would be a dramatically life changing event. For Mom, it was just another trip to the hospital to get her body back into shape. Mom and Dad became familiar with how to live comfortably with an ostomy bag. Basically, Mom's life was back to regular; visiting with friends, shopping with Dad, and volunteering next door at the church keeping the altar tidy and decorated with flowers. After more than a year with the ostomy bag, the surgeon said it was time for Mom to come back to the hospital and have her bowels put back together. This worked well; however, the bowel was a bit shorter from then on.

Late spring or early summer of 1994 the story begins to change. With the shorter bowel, it was common for Mom to have long bouts of loose stool. To treat this, Mom had a little tablet that helped slow the flow through her body. One sunny morning Mom was having this issue, so she took a tablet to help slow the flow. This didn't help so she took another tablet. After about four hours she had taken over five of these tablets and it was not helping.

On the other hand, she was progressively becoming lethargic, weak and her ankles were swelling. Unfortunately, Mom had mistaken her diarrhea pills for her heart medication. They were both small round tablets and Mom had the tendency to take tablets based upon the color and shape of the tablet rather than the name written on the label of the bottle. Over the course of 4-5 hours Mom had accidently been inducing congestive heart failure upon herself, thinking she was treating her diarrhea.

Dad called 911 and Mom was once again taken to the hospital. After a few days in the intensive care unit, she was stabilized and then released home. This was really hard on her heart as well as the rest of her body. She was tired. Over the next few days all of our family came to Mt. Shasta to say goodbye to Mom. Hospice was called in and before long Mom passed peacefully in her sleep.

12

Geographical

Please understand, I was secretly using an increasing number of opiates and cocaine over the past three years. This addiction was increasingly controlling my life. In addition, my drug use was overwhelmingly impacting our spiritual, emotional, and physical family life through all of this. Unfortunately, I was the only one who knew about this and was positive I had it all under control.

Before Mom passed, we had already decided that we were going to move back to Santa Cruz. We were looking for a home that had a studio attached to it so Mom and Dad could move with us. Deep inside my brain, I felt that if I was able to move from one geographical location to another, I would be able to start all over and not need to use drugs anymore. Of course, as we know, addiction doesn't work that way.

Our plans were to move to Santa Cruz, and I would become the Director of Pharmacy for the newly built Sutter Hospital. The opening day was still about a year out so I would practice at the local Medical Clinic Pharmacy for the time being. I was to start at the beginning of July; however, we had not yet sold our house in Mt. Shasta. With delusions of a life I would never see until I stopped doing drugs, I packed up and moved to Santa Cruz to live with my sister Lydia. In Mt. Shasta I had left my loving and devoted wife, two amazing children at one and three years old, and my Dad who had moved in with Susie and the kids.

The goal was to find a house to rent, bring the family down, and sell the house in Mt. Shasta. This was a long couple of months. Thinking back at the discomfort, pain and loneliness Susie must have felt creates a sense of regret deep in my soul. She paid the bills, managed the house with the kids, and packed all of our belongings in preparation for the time when I found a house for them to come down to.

Finally, I was able to find us a small two bedroom home down toward the end of 26th avenue, one block back from the beach. My plan was to drive up to Mt. Shasta on Friday after work with my friend, rent a U-Haul truck on Saturday and start packing, finish packing Sunday morning and drive back to Santa Cruz. Realistically, I should have planned for a week off work and a team of helpers to come do the packing; however, I was on a mission and was sure I could handle it.

We got the U-Haul packed, Kendyl and our dog Rolff in the U-Haul with me while Susie and Cooper were in the mustang. My friend took off ahead with his van also packed with our belongings. It was late in the afternoon when we finally got on the road and the six hour drive back to Santa Cruz had never seemed longer. Unfortunately, I was coming down from whatever I had been taking the previous week and was absolutely bleary eyed sleepy. By the time we got to Los Gatos I needed to pull over on the side of the road and rest my eyes for 30 minutes. Not a fun trip.

We pulled into our rental in Santa Cruz sometime around 10pm. To have something to sleep on I needed to open the back of the U-Haul and drag out one of our mattresses to put on the living room floor with some blankets and sleeping bags. Yes, it was a cute home; however, it was small, and neighbors were right next door on both sides. This was a far cry from the acre of property and custom home we had been living in up in Mt. Shasta. Once again, I had made a life changing decision that affected the entire family, without giving Susie an opportunity to share how it made her feel or even whether she wanted any of it.

Bless her heart, she made it into a home. The next few months we settled into a somewhat peaceful routine of Santa Cruz life. I was working 10-hour days, five days a week (sometimes Saturdays as well); however,

Susie would do her best to have dinner ready for us when I got home. We would work with the kids, get them to bed, and continue to move forward with the life we were living. During this same time, Dad moved back to Santa Cruz and was able to rent a home near my sister's house on the other side of town..

Through it all was this undercurrent that I knew needed to be addressed; however, there was absolutely no way I could ever talk about it. My drug use was increasing. Evidently, moving to another geographical location is not enough to change the addiction. It will get better, in about 18 months or so, but first we need to move to another house.

13

Our Home

Emotions were beginning to boil. Along with rent on our home in Santa Cruz, we still owned our house in Mt. Shasta. This was a recession and our home in Mt. Shasta had lost nearly 20% of its value. We had it for sale for over six months and not one offer. We needed to rent the house in order to maintain some sort of income to help pay the mortgage.

Our realtor helped us find a tenant; however, we soon realized our new renter was less than honest in her approach to managing fiscal manners. Not only were we not receiving rent, but we also needed to move through the eviction process from 400 miles away.

Sometime around March, after living in the beach house for six months, Susie found us a home. She was driving down Brommer street and saw a for sale sign in the ground on a hill in front of the oldest and largest Victorian farmhouse in Live Oak. Looking at the property from across the street, it looked amazing. Tall two-story Victorian framing, big front porch, and property that stood 10 feet up above the road down below. Covered in fruit trees, flowers and roses, Susie fell in love with it right away. She had a way of seeing the immense future potential of this house.

On the other hand, as we walked up the driveway and got closer to the house, we could see that the entire front of the house was covered with aluminum siding to cover the damaged wood that was behind it. All around the sides and back of the house we could see the green chipping paint and cracked boards. As well, the 37 single pane windows and hollow walls did little to insulate the home from the cold fog air that surrounded the sleeping giant of a house.

Walking through the house for the first time, what comes to mind is the number of doors. Each and every room could be closed off from all of the other rooms by closing doors. Living room, kitchen, dining room, entry room, everything; all doors. In addition, the entire house was heated by one floor grate furnace that was in the front living room. None of this mattered to Susie, she could see through all of it and had a vision. I'm not sure she knew exactly what that vision was; however, it was strong with emotion, and she wanted this house.

The property was large to match the house, nearly one full acre. Perhaps the entire project gave Susie a sense of control over her life, a control that I had been slowly retracting from her over the past three years. I agreed that this would be our home and we proceeded to try and figure out a way to purchase the property. Over the years Susie has helped me understand how easily a project may flow when all the pieces come into alignment; as well, she has shown me how difficult a project may become when barriers get in our way. Unfortunately, I have not always been aware of the barriers and continued to push through when it would have been more appropriate to step back and re-evaluate.

For example, as I described earlier, when we were purchasing our first home in Mt. Shasta, our realtor helped us with the down payment and the process was ultra-smooth. Contrary to our first purchase, our move to our fancy second home in Mt. Shasta was not so smooth. We came up against financial barriers which needed to be surmounted and the end result was a lingering discomfort. Of course, yes, some of that discomfort was my unresolved drug addiction; however, the discomfort was definitely a sign that we should have taken a step back and evaluated our choices.

The purchase of our Brommer street home was smooth. Susie and I still owned our home in Mt. Shasta, and we had a difficult time keeping a paying tenant in the home while we waited for a buyer to come along. To my recollection, the rent we received paid about one-fifth of our monthly fees on the home.

With all this in mind, we had our real estate agent approach the seller's agent and see if we could come up with a deal. With grace on our side, the owners agreed to sell us the home with no down payment. In addition, they agreed to carry a four year, interest only, loan for us. They really appreciated that a young family was moving in and was planning on making this their home. Their one request was that we please make it our home rather than demolishing the house and building a cul-de-sac of three or four homes on the property.

In April of 1995, we moved into our new home. This was an incredibly exciting time. Susie and I had come together, worked as a team, and purchased our home in Santa Cruz. We both knew this was going to be tremendous amounts of work; however, we had done this before with our first home we purchased seven years earlier. In our married life of just under seven years we had already lived in three houses and were moving into our 4th. We both agreed that living in an old home that we create as our own was our preference.

At this time, it would have been appropriate for Susie and me to obtain the help of a seasoned home remodeler in order to define how we should proceed over the next couple years. Instead, we had the inside of the house painted, cleaned up the bathroom, tore up some old carpet, took off some of the excess doors, moved in and continued our life.

The kids loved it. The house was big with old floors and was great for roller skating. We had this loop that went from the front room, through the kitchen, into our bedroom, past the bathroom and back through the living room into the front room. Kendyl would skate, Cooper would run and Rolff, our black lab, would bark.

Even though the house was big, we created our bedrooms all next to each other. Susie and I had a room right off the kitchen and Cooper and Kendyl each had rooms that were connected to our bedroom. The house had been remodeled multiple times over the previous 100 years (built in

1895) and the current arrangement of rooms didn't necessarily make much sense. The upstairs was a separate 2-bedroom apartment that needed renovation so for the meantime, we just used the space as storage.

I wish I could say that we moved in, created our life, and lived happily ever after; however, that's not quite how this story goes. I know Susie was doing the best she could with what she had. The house was a huge project just to make it comfortable for her and the kids. In addition, she would spend time out in the yard, playing with the kids and teaching them about gardening and digging in the dirt.

We would work on trying to create time for each other, to do things with friends or have some reason to get out on our own; however, my self-centered behavior kept getting in the way. Unfortunately, I was still under the impression that I had everything under control. We were managing two mortgages, while I continued to work more than 50 hours per week. In addition, I was becoming increasingly unavailable both physically and emotionally with my secret drug addiction.

14

Truth

It was my intention to stop using drugs and become the husband I knew my wife deserved; however, I couldn't. Many times, I tried, for six or 24 hours. Each time ended abruptly. The thought of telling Susie was absolutely incomprehensible. If I did, I was sure I would lose absolutely everything. If I didn't, my fear is that I would die before I could apologize for creating such a frantic mess of her life. Backed into the corner, I continued to use and portray the image that I had everything in complete control.

During this time, we would still go to church on a semi-regular basis. This one morning, 3/10/96, only 11 months after moving into our new home, I went to Sunday service at Star of the Sea catholic church on my own, while Susie stayed home with Cooper and Kendyl. This Sunday morning was a packed house. I remember sitting somewhere in the middle and listening to Father Rene's homily. He was talking about Mary at the well in the middle of a hot summer day.

Being that this was nearly three decades ago, without paraphrasing exactly, I'll do my best at the story. Jesus was walking along and came to this well around noon. He saw this young lady and was asking her why she was at the well in the heat of the midday sun. She stumbled with her answer, and he said it was ok, she didn't need to answer, he already knew why she was there. Jesus went on to tell her that he knew she was there at noon because she was too ashamed to come out in the early cool morning when all of the other ladies would be there. Jesus went on to explain that he understood she was unable to face the other ladies because she had been sleeping with all of their husbands.

The young lady, a little dumbfounded that this guy would know about all of this, just stood there not sure what to do. Jesus then took her by the hand and had her walk into town with him. He let her know they were going to go to all of the homes of these people, and she would apologize to the families for her part in the inappropriate behavior. Jesus assured her it would all be ok if she just allowed him to lead her through the process.

Here's where the story gets interesting. Father Rene then looked out into the entire congregation of what must have been over 200 people. I felt him look directly at me, as if what he was about to say was meant specifically for me to hear. He said that today is the day we go home and take care of any issue that we have been lying about. Don't delay, do it right away. The message seemed incredibly clear to me. Somehow, I have been given a chance to break free and importantly, freely accept the consequences that would be dealt to me.

Throughout my sober life I have come to recognize miracles. Miracles exist all around us, each and every day. Prior to this moment I didn't really have an understanding of what that meant. How could it be that something was out there that happened without me having an understanding of how or why it was happening. After I entered a new way of living, it became clear and ever so obvious to me that miracles had been happening all around me throughout my life; Susie, Cooper, and Kendyl for starters. Up and till this point, I couldn't recognize a miracle if it was staring me in the face.

After church that morning I went directly home and let Susie know we needed to talk. We sat at the dining room table and without delay I told her that I am a drug addict. While my momentum was rolling, I continued on and explained that I had a vial of cocaine in my briefcase, had been drinking hydrocodone cough syrup on a regular basis, and that I had been stealing these drugs from my employer. This was miracle number one. How, today, was I able to sit in front of my dear wife who I had been lying to for the past few years and tell her all of this? This was no power of my own. I had experienced a miracle of grace, come down into me, and carried me through the past 60 minutes.

Honestly, Susie's initial reaction was relief. She knew I had not been present mentally or physically with her for quite some time now and she had concerns that perhaps I was having an affair. Of course, and rightly so, her initial reaction of relief promptly changed to anger when she realized the gravity of what was unfolding in front of her. This anger was immediately followed by fear of what would happen to her and the kids as a consequence of my negligent behavior.

We cried. We knew from this moment on everything was going to change. It was clear that I could not live the lie any longer. My job at this moment was to let the truth out and accept the consequences. After our initial conversation around the dining room table, we called the owner of the pharmacy that I had been working at. Without giving him much of a chance to say anything I let it all out, telling him I was using drugs, stealing them from the store, and was ready to accept what was coming to me. Being the gracious and loving man that he was, he said he would meet me at the store, and we would call the California State Board of Pharmacy Pharmacists Recovery Program and ask for help.

The following 24 hours were filled with tears as I let my Dad, sisters and brothers know what was happening. Over the past two years I had told lies to just about everyone I had come in contact with. My stories were grandiose and indisputable, mainly due to the fact that I was unable to engage anyone in an honest conversation about reality. I can recall lying in bed that night next to Susie, feeling the penetrating physical angst of an addict in need of drugs while also an incredible spiritual lightness that only comes from complete and utter honesty.

Just to reiterate, my employer could have called the sheriff and had me arrested for stealing thousands of dollars' worth of drugs from the pharmacy. Instead, he helped me call the state board of pharmacy and ask for help. This is definitely another miracle. The following morning, I woke up and was really beginning to feel uncomfortable in my skin. All I could think of was how I was feeling physically and how I was going to fix this. I was in the kitchen alone, reached into the cabinet and found the only bottle of alcohol we currently had in the house, a bottle of Bailey's Irish Cream. As per my normal secret way of life, I looked around the corners to make sure no one was watching, opened the bottle and took a couple of long draws. This was my last use of either drugs or alcohol, the morning of 3/11/96.

15

Alcoholic – Addict

For me, and many other alcoholics or addicts, drugs and alcohol start as a simple mechanism for changing how we are feeling. It's not necessarily something that is obvious, we just happen to have a social drink some time in our early life and WOW, the world seems just a little more attainable. We don't consciously attempt to disguise our emotions so we may be more likable, it just happens that when we drink, we find ourselves feeling a little more outgoing and maybe a little less shy. It becomes a learned behavior.

This is certainly not the case for everyone; however, you may recognize this behavior. Maybe we have a difficult time talking with groups of people and find that after a few drinks we become more sociable. Unfortunately, we don't realize that with proper tools and intervention, we could uncover what causes our shyness. Then, with a little effort, we might learn some communication tools so we may better express ourselves. Instead, we find with just a few drinks of alcohol, we are able to loosen up, tell stories and make people laugh.

As we grow older, our emotions begin to run a bit deeper and become integrally entwined with our ever-growing responsibilities. We have school to complete, jobs to show up at, families to provide for and an ever-increasing amount of bills we are responsible for paying. Fortunately, our brain remembers how to subdue and control all of these insidious emotions that continually want to express themselves. Our learned behavior.

Remember when we had that first beer? Remember how loose and awesome it made us feel? I do.

***

Throughout my 18 years of drinking and using drugs, from the fall of 1977 through the spring of 1996, I was on a slow exponential curve. My heart is telling me I need to discuss how it felt, emotionally, rather than dive deep into all of the stories that happened due to drugs and alcohol during this time. My fear in telling specific stories is that I may somehow glamorize the hipness and coolness of using drugs in an effort to minimize the gravity of what was happening. This is one of the tools of life I would regularly use; the glamorization of inappropriate behavior in order to minimize the perceived negative consequences.

Rather, I will take a small number of carefully crafted words to do my best at describing what my addiction was like and where it came from.

When I was in high school, on weekends I drank to get drunk. I was shy and alcohol helped me get over my self-perceived awkwardness in social situations. Beer, liquor, it didn't matter. It was not uncommon for me to get so drunk that I would black out and not remember what I did the night before. Multiple times I would drive drunk, the window rolled down, my hand over one eye so I wasn't seeing double vision and take the backroads home to avoid police.

On the other hand, I was on the honor roll, applied to college, senior class president, participated in sports, and worked 20 hours per week at the local grocery store. My impression was that I was totally under control.

During my six years of college, I continued to drink to get drunk on weekends, while also adding in a few weeknights here and there. As well, I began smoking marijuana on a weekly basis, sometimes daily. I experimented with cocaine, mushrooms, and benzodiazepines. The feeling I got from cocaine was complete control; however, it was expensive. I was able to position myself maybe six or seven times during college where I was given cocaine. My tolerance to alcohol and ability to hide my drug use and drinking, as well as my ability to masquerade my emotions, grew exponentially throughout these years.

Correspondingly, I maintained multiple highly functional intern pharmacist positions, ran in 10K races on a regular basis, was named California Society of Hospital Pharmacists student of the year, functioned as a student advisor to incoming pharmacy students, and graduated pharmacy school on the deans' honor roll. Again, it was my impression that I was in complete control and that I could stop any time I wanted.

As a practicing pharmacist, I steadily increased my use of opiates, cocaine, and benzodiazepines over the course of seven years. My emotional availability to a loving family drifted as I became overwhelmingly consumed in self-centered behaviors. I worked hard to try and cover up my advancing addiction. Late nights and early mornings at work, extra shifts, overtime whenever possible; these diversions were all just a counterbalance to throw off any suspecting coworkers or family members. How could a loved one, who works so diligently, possibly be doing anything unethical or immoral? My misguided intelligence led me to believe I had everything under control. Inappropriate logic leads me, a highly-functioning addict, to think everything is just fine as long as I continue to thrive successfully at work and maintain family responsibilities. I neglected to notice the slow deterioration of my physical, mental, emotional, and spiritual health. My wife, co-workers and family members began to show real concern; however, I became very comfortable with not telling the truth.

During those seven years, I practiced pharmacy in a hospital setting, performed clinical consults on a daily basis, developed policies and procedures for regulatory accreditation, participated in multiple code-blue situations and worked my way into a hospital pharmacy management position. In addition, I got married, had two children, and moved my family three times.

The path I was on was getting steeper and increasingly more unpredictable. The further my pendulum swung into my addiction, the more strenuous and diligent my work would become to balance the powerful counter swing. Not much longer and I am certain I would have ended up either in an institution or dead.

Not many options exist for an individual who has come to this point. The fear of being found out is incomprehensible. Many will continue on in denial until they are caught up in a lie with the authorities and find themselves in jail. Others will continue until their bodies won't tolerate another day and find themselves in a hospital. Those of us saved by an intervention are the fortunate. Be it divine or friends and family, the result is the same, treatment and recovery. With divine intervention, and the assistance of a loving wife, boss, and family, I entered a drug and alcohol treatment program in March of 1996.

16

Recovery

My brother came over about noon to pick me up and drive to the recovery center, less than two miles from our home. I entered the doors at Janus of Santa Cruz and took the first step toward a new life.

Janus of Santa Cruz has two separate recovery spaces. Downstairs is a detox unit where addicts and alcoholics can stay for up to seven days, depending upon their situation. If everything goes well during the detox portion of your stay, then you may qualify to be moved upstairs to the 28-day treatment program. Vividly I can remember walking into the office of the detox unit and sitting in a chair next to a counselor. Still, it didn't really dawn on me exactly what was happening. Just a couple days before I had been working behind the counter in a professional pharmacy, serving patients, consulting with physicians. Now, here I am, sitting in this smelly and musty space, waiting to be admitted into a detox unit with a bunch of drunks and junkies.

Not having any sober tools, I was still using the only tools I knew; talk quickly, be the first to comment, correct anyone who says something wrong, and act like the smartest person in the room. These tools had done well for me over the past years; however, I could soon tell it wasn't going to work here. As someone once told me, now is the time to take the cotton out of my ears and put it in my mouth. This was my absolute first exposure to alcoholics anonymous. Up until this point, I had no idea of how to stop using cocaine, opiates, benzodiazepines, marijuana, or alcohol.

That first evening in Janus I went to my first AA meeting. There was a gentleman named Bill. He was a physician in Santa Cruz. He came in to tell his story of what happened while he was using, how he got sober, and what it is like now. He went on to describe how he used drugs at work, regularly. He would be in the room next to his patients getting loaded, then just go back to work. He explained exactly what I felt; we are professional health care providers. We have studied and trained and are at the top of our game. We know what we are taking and we, above all others, know exactly how to control it. We know exactly how to stop and can stop whenever we need to.

He then went on to describe how it got out of control. Maybe he would wake up with a hangover and go directly to the freezer and take a pull of cold vodka to relax the pain in his brain. His family was falling apart because of the regular stream of lies he was telling to cover up his daily and nightly drinking and drugging. Furthermore, he went on to describe his deteriorating physical and spiritual health, all the while confident he had everything still completely under control.

He stated, in a self-revealing way that made a huge impact on me, that he was so incredibly grateful that he was pulled over, arrested, and taken to jail for drunk driving. This was his impactful moment. He went on to learn about AA, gain gratitude for life and an understanding of emotions, and learn how to live life sober.

Up until this very moment, I had no idea that other people were going through what I had been going through. This gentleman, in the course of a 30-minute story, was able to very closely describe how my life had been unfolding over the past four years, and then give me a glimpse of where my life may go from here if I just pay attention, take advice, and practice gratitude.

***

After a few days in the detox unit, I was qualified to be moved up stairs to the 28-day treatment program. What an incredibly interesting world I was entering. Many treatment facilities have lovely grounds to walk around, plenty of personal time, exercise rooms and swimming pools, group discussions and plenty of classes on how to live a sober life. For some inexplicable reason, the facility near our home was absolutely none of those.

Janus of Santa Cruz is a cement building in a residential block. The redeeming factor is that it is just one block away from the beach. I wasn't moving into some Betty Ford clinic with well-to-do alcoholics and office working drug addicts. Interestingly, this recovery center was based on giving anyone and everyone a chance for recovery. Less than fortunate and disenfranchised individuals down on their financial luck, along with a few homeless individuals who had a run in with the legal system and chose rehab over jail were my roommates for the next month.

The entry date into the program was rolling. In other words, the day I entered the program just happened to be the graduation for someone else who had completed the 28 days. There was no particular start date each month, you just entered the program when you did and then 28 days later you graduated, assuming you completed the entire program. The facility housed about 25 individuals, and just about every time someone left, a new person would come in and start the program.

Quite often, two of the main items missing in an alcoholics' life are schedule and accountability. Life in this particular recovery facility does its best to help its residents understand the importance of both showing up on time as well as taking responsibility for our actions.

The program consisted of group sessions, lots of writing, 12-step meeting attendance and some individual counseling; however, the main aspect of the entire 28 days was truth.

This program worked on the idea that anyone who breaks the rules during their stay at Janus needs to leave immediately. The rules are clear and reviewed on a daily basis. The catch is, there are no counselors staying in the building with us. The only time we see counselors is during group sessions. The rest of the approximately 20 hours per day are utilized just living with your recovery people.

There is this strange self-governance cycle that works through the facility. The senior residents show the newbies how the program works so that when the newbies become senior residents, they can be the teachers. The chores, such as cleaning the restrooms, kitchen and great room, sweeping the front entrance, and managing the cleaning roster change each week. Initially, a resident will have a straightforward job like mopping the bathroom. The jobs change each week. By the fourth week, a resident may be responsible for managing the cleaning load of four other residents. Again, this is all part of understanding the importance of showing up and maintaining accountability.

Along with growing one's own personal accountability and responsibility, residents are required to share with the group when they have encountered one of the other residents engaging in inappropriate behavior. This is the quintessential center of accountability. Each resident is responsible for discussing with the group when they recognize another resident who is not following the rules.

For example, the rules were specific against any sort of inappropriate fraternization between residents, no leaving the facility after hours, no walking outside of the designated areas, no leaving on a walk without at least three residents in the group, and a host of other rules. Everyone was aware of and had more than enough opportunity to familiarize themselves with the rules.

The issue is, many of the residents were here, specifically, because they felt rules didn't apply to them. In addition to those who broke the rules, it was imperative for the individual who saw them, to speak up at group and bring it to the attention of everyone, including the counselors.

We, as humans, are conditioned somehow to just look the other way when we see something inappropriate happening. By doing this we are being complicit in inappropriate activity or action. The goal of this recovery center is to teach individuals how to not only become accountable for their own actions, but to also take responsibility in maintaining the rules of the institution in order to help everyone live in a safe and caring environment.

Of course, during the process of group sessions and homework we learn a myriad of tools to implement in order to help us maintain a sober lifestyle. Being new to recovery, I didn't realize how often individuals would relapse and start using again. About halfway through the program one of the counselors said that if all of us were still sober one year from today he would take us all out to dinner at the Chaminade restaurant. To me, this sounded crazy because he was looking at about $2000 to feed us all at that place. What I didn't realize at the time was that it was nearly guaranteed that all 25 of us would not be sober 12 months from now. After 12 months, I was the only one who was still sober.

So, the first miracle I talked about, a few pages back, is when, of no power of my own, I walked into the house, sat down with Susie, and let her know I am a drug addict and alcoholic.

This next miracle I am about to describe is no less dramatic. After about two weeks in the facility, I had a visit from the California State Board of Pharmacy inspector. During my discussion with him I wanted to assure that the owner of the store had no idea that I had been taking drugs and that it was definitely all my fault. We had a very friendly discussion, and he did quite a bit of documenting.

Before he left, he shared with me that the store I was working at had shown up on his radar as a store of concern due to the large amounts of controlled substances that had been purchased over the past 12 months. He went on to let me know that a sting operation had been placed on the calendar and had I not serendipitously turned myself in, he would have visited the store in the very near future with a sheriff. Most likely I would have been led out of the store in handcuffs and taken to jail.

17

Real Life

Here I was, living in an institution, which was basically a hotel, for a month. All my meals are taken care of, and I spend my day talking and sharing with people. The goal was to make it through the 28-day program and then graduate with tools to take home and begin a new sober life. While I was doing this, Susie was living at home, with our two-year-old son and four-year-old daughter.

It's difficult to imagine, or even put into words, what Susie must have been going through. Of course, she supported me emotionally and very much wished for me to get help. On the other hand, we had purchased this home in Santa Cruz 12 months earlier and we still owned our home in Mt. Shasta. Here she was, two mortgages to pay, and her husband is in drug rehab. Furthermore, this was a relatively cold March, and the house had yet to have any renovations completed. Our sole source of heat was a floor furnace in the front room. I can picture her wrapping blankets around her two lovely children and holding them while snuggling on the couch in the only room that had any heat.

After four long weeks I returned home to my family. Both Susie and the kids were incredibly happy to have me back home; however, life had changed. Everything we had known would now be a little different. Communication, truth, understanding, listening; it all had to be on the table. It wasn't as if I could just waltz back in the house and ask my family to trust me. This is an incredibly long process, and I wasn't in the position to rush it with any of them.

After the welcome home happiness, Susie and I had to have the important discussion of how we were going to pay for life. Susie had done a tremendous job of keeping the house together over the past four weeks, as well as the past few years. Fortunately, when I had just begun my career as a pharmacist, I had purchased a disability insurance policy. This policy, once approved, paid half of my annual salary until I was able to step back into a pharmacy and continue to practice again. As well, Susie completed her resume and went looking for a job. With her medical office experience, she quickly landed a position working for a local plastic surgeon running the front office. I know this had not been in her plan, needing to go back to work before her kid's started kindergarten; however, Susie believed in our core family and we both wanted to make this work.

Over the previous few years, I had been creating an increasingly chaotic and uncomfortable dynamic in our household. This ever-increasing chaos had moved Susie into action as a controller of the house. She did an excellent job of bringing together the complexities of household function as well as loving childcare. This was being completed during a disturbing amount of dysfunction from her husband. The more dysfunction I brought into and around the family and house, the more she stepped up to manage the environment. During the last couple months prior to my sobriety date Susie had stepped into a full-on crisis management role, doing her best to shield and protect herself and our children from my erratic and disruptive behavior.

After I got back from rehab we needed, as a family, to slowly come to the understanding that we were not in crisis mode. Our path had changed; however, I was the only one who had left and gone through treatment. Susie and the kids had been at home, managing the crisis and working out their own way of coping with me being gone. When I returned, the house was ready for disruption to come back; however, I was now holding still. My wife and children had been conditioned to expect an unsettling disturbance every time I walked through the door; however, the crisis had been mitigated and there was currently not any turmoil to control. We just needed time and hours and hours of talking.

***

Here's some important details to meditate on. For the 12 or more months leading up to me entering rehab, I was becoming increasingly manipulative and dishonest. Multiple times my siblings and my Dad would point out that I didn't seem quite right. They would beat around the bush a little; however, their question was always of concern for my well-being. They just felt something was off and weren't exactly sure how to describe it. I was always very clear in my answers that it was just a stressful time in my life. We currently owned two houses, I was working more than 50 hours each week, and the home we were living in needed extensive renovation. I presented myself in what felt like a genuine and authentic manner, and it appeared they believed my lie.

On the other hand, Susie was certain something was off. She was living with a complete lunatic and absolutely no one would listen to her. She saw that I would regularly make up excuses to go back to the pharmacy after I had come home from work. I would spend time alone out in the shed under the premise that I needed some alone time to work on my projects. I would stay up to all hours of the night and then sleep in until just before I needed to jump out of bed and get to work. She saw that my weight had increased to more than 220 pounds and I had all but given up on exercising. On a regular basis she would notice that I was sweating, just sitting still in the living room or at the dining room table. In addition, my ability to perform sexually had decreased down to zero. It was commonplace that I wasn't present emotionally for conversations or to work through household, not to mention personal issues.

Susie would have talks with her and my family. They would advise to just hold on, things will get better. She would be told that maybe if she had dinner ready for me when I got home from my busy stressful day at work, that might help smooth things out. Just keep managing the household, do the shopping, keep the yard put together, take care of the kids all day every day, make breakfast and dinner and a lunch to go, keep the kitchen clean, have all the clothes washed and pharmacy shirts ironed, have the kids bathed and fed, and maybe put on something nice before Steve gets home so he can see how pretty you are. In other words, suck it up girl, you got a good life. It's not every wife who gets to stay home with the kids while your dear husband goes off to work every day. Stop complaining and blaming Steve because you're having trouble making things work.

My wife is my rock. She is absolutely the best thing that has ever happened to me. Through all of this she stayed strong and held the family together. Even more, after I came home from rehab, she worked with me, on a daily basis, to build our relationship. Believe me, this was not easy. We had many nights where we talked for hours, tears, anger, resentment, confusion, and love. The difference now is that we were both being truthful and authentic in our conversations. This was a new life for us and our core group, me, Susie, Kendyl, and Cooper were the focus of our life. We had a very small circle that we interacted with. Slowly over the years we expanded our circle of relations; however, at the slightest moment, we would pull back to just four in order to maintain our family.

***

As Susie returned to work, my life soon became very busy in a once-in-a-life-time way. First and foremost, I was now a stay-at-home dad with a soon to be three-year-old and five-year-old. The gift of being present for children, participating in their life, at their level, is absolutely wonderful. Kendyl was just finishing up her first year at pre-school and would be moving on to kindergarten the following year. Cooper was preparing to start pre-school the following year so he would come with me to drop Kendyl off at pre-school and then in the afternoon to pick her up.

My first couple months sober, after taking Susie to work, Cooper and I would walk Kendyl down to the Family Network preschool. What a treat this was, packing up Kendyl for the day, and walking with her to school. Cooper and I would walk in with her and spend one or two minutes visiting just to make sure she made it there and got settled. I remember the teacher telling me one time that Kendyl had this special way about her. Whenever anyone new started at the school, Kendyl would graciously make them feel welcome by introducing herself and then proceeding to show them where everything was located.

On the walk back home Cooper and I had this thing where we would look up at a certain set of trees. There was this vacant property along the way that had a grove of tall ancient Bay trees. These trees are messy and have peeling bark and stringy leaves hanging all around them. In a grove, the peeling bark appears to jump from tree to tree. To Cooper and me, this looked like a tree full of snakes. We would always be looking up to see if the snakes were moving.

During the day we would do our best to manage the house as well as Susie had done, quickly realizing how difficult it was to organize all the chores and keep everything kept and tidy. I soon found out that I was relatively good at keeping things tidy; however, maintaining a clean household, I came to find out, was entirely different than keeping it tidy.

We would try to get through the laundry, keep up on the dishes, brush our hair and make our beds. The kids could tell, this might be kind of fun having dad home like this for a while; however, it wasn't mom. We did our best, and every day around 5pm we would all get in the car and drive down to pick up Susie from work. Yes, at the time we were living with one car, and it was common for us to all get in the car and drive Susie to work in the morning and then go pick her up in the afternoon.

It was during this time that I also began to work on my recovery. For quite a few years I was a regular, at least five days per week, at AA or NA meetings. I found a sponsor and proceeded to work through the 12 steps.

As a condition of my voluntary participation in the pharmacist's recovery program I was required to attend a weekly health professional recovery group as well as weekly therapy with a private counselor. In addition, every single morning I needed to phone into a message machine at the state board of pharmacy to see if I needed to go and have a urine test done that day. There was no pattern at all to the testing; however, overall, I was called in to test about once every three weeks.

Quite often we would pack up and go meet my sister with her day-care kids at the Frederick Street park for a play date or go visit my Dad at his house and talk and play for a couple hours. Dad had a neat little house near the Grant Street park, and he was always more than happy to go for a walk with us to go play for a while. As well, my sister's house always had plenty of toys in the back yard and two or three kids to play with.

Just a couple months into sobriety I had a doctor's appointment at the Santa Cruz Medical Clinic on Soquel Avenue. This was a day that Susie had off from work, and it is less than two miles to the clinic, so I decided to walk down for my appointment. Following the appointment, I was walking home through Arana Gulch, on the dirt trail before it was paved, looking out over the harbor and the ocean. At that point in time, I remember thinking how rich I was.

My spiritual being had given me the opportunity to live a sober life, and along with it came an understanding of authenticity and truth. Financially we were about as tight as we had ever been. Every five dollar bill was accounted for and put toward either food or bills. The richness I was experiencing at that point in time is not a feeling that can be purchased with money. I had my life, health, and love of my family. In addition, I was living in this amazingly beautiful location and was incredibly excited to see what each and every day was going to surprise me with.

18

Addiction Counseling School

At 32 years old, married with two children, I was unsure if I was ever going to be allowed to practice pharmacy again. Susie and I needed to come up with a plan. Currently, Susie was working at the medical clinic, and I was receiving disability payments from my private insurance I had purchased seven years prior; however, this would not suffice as our sustainable future plan. After much thought and discussion, we decided I would utilize what I already know. We created a plan that I would use my knowledge of medications as well as my understanding of drugs from an addict's perspective and become a drug and alcohol counselor.

We found a one-year certification program in addiction counseling offered at Bethany College in Scotts Valley. This course fit into our schedule with classes on Friday nights from 6-10pm and all-day Saturdays from 9-5. This schedule would allow me to be present for the kids all week long while Susie worked while also giving me some direction to focus my scattered energy.

During the week I would get up and be at an AA meeting at 6am on a daily basis. As well, I would participate in group therapy with other pharmacists, doctors, and dentists every Wednesday evening. In addition, I would attend private therapy with a licensed counselor every Tuesday afternoon. As if this wasn't enough for me to help understand myself, I was immersed in drug and alcohol counseling class every Friday night and all-day Saturday.

Come to find out, counseling school is pretty much like going to therapy, only much more intense. First of all, every person in the addiction counseling program was also at some stage of recovery themselves. This created an environment such that every class session had the feel of a group AA or therapy session. Next, it seemed that every topic I was discussing in my therapy sessions was reviewed in class that week. As well, topics we discussed in class seemed to work their way into my therapy sessions for the following week. They not only enhanced each other; it seemed as if one always led into the next in a serendipitously obvious manner.

***

One of the first major topics discussed in our addiction counseling program was the tool of creating a timeline. The idea is to truthfully document your drinking or using history. When was your first drink? When did you first black out? When did you start using marijuana, hard alcohol, and other drugs? When did the using begin affecting your physical and spiritual health? How and when did alcohol or drug use affect your personal relationships or work life? As you can imagine, this is quite a lengthy project and may take multiple hours over a couple weeks in order to do a complete and thorough timeline. Quite often it takes the help of someone else working with you to help genuinely complete the timeline.

My timeline began in counseling class, and then I talked about it with Susie, then I took it to therapy, and finally I talked about it with my health care professional group. Again, I kept doing this circle of presenting my timeline and communicating until we all agreed we had an understanding of the cycle of events. Throughout the process a theme kept recurring which I have referred to previously a few pages back. My life, from the time I entered high school, until I entered recovery, was on an ever-increasing pendulum. I was a people pleaser, plain and simple. Throughout high school I was engaged, participated, performed and did well. On the other hand, I realized how wonderful it was to get black out drunk and not have a care. Through college my participation grew

106

stronger and my need to succeed to show everyone I could do it was a leading factor in my success. As well, I absolutely loved smoking dope and spending time by myself in my own little world away from everyone and everything. Through the first seven years of my professional life my desire to show everyone how quickly I could become successful in my career was a demanding task that took everything I could give. On the other hand, more than ever, I just wanted to lock myself in the garage by myself and get loaded.

The further the pendulum swung to one side, the further it would need to swing back the other way to balance itself out. Now and again, for a fleeting few moments, the pendulum would be suspended either at the top of one side, the top of the other, or just straight up and down. For a snapshot in time, that went away as quickly as it was noticed, the world would feel right. These snapshots grew further and further apart to the point where they felt completely unobtainable.

***

Initially, in my humble opinion, we use alcohol or drugs to change how we feel. Like I was discussing earlier, our inhibitions may be decreased, and we become the person we think we want to be. Sometimes this may advance beyond who we think we want to be, and we might hurt someone else emotionally, act incredibly inappropriate or perform reckless and illegal behavior. We don't see this coming and may not even realize it as it is happening; however, at some point the drug and alcohol use changes from simply changing how we feel, to daily use.

Addiction doesn't necessarily just all of a sudden happen. Over the course of weeks, months or even years we slowly increase our use as our family, work, physical and mental health slowly deteriorate. Without even realizing it, we are at a point where every day we need to use drugs or alcohol in order to keep from going into withdrawals and getting sick.

Physiologically, our body produces endorphins in response to physical or mental stress. These endorphins are utilized to help fight our own pain and to help us make appropriate decisions during stressful situations.

Any addict will tell you about how amazing it feels, both physically and mentally, to treat their sickness with an opiate or a drink of their favorite alcoholic beverage. The clouds clear from the brain, smooth soft emotions roll over their body, and all is right with the world once again. Until that point, absolutely nothing else matters. Every cell in your body is craving the next use. The trouble is, it is short lived and will soon need to be treated once again.

As I said, our body makes its own endorphins. When we ingest opiates, and to some degree alcohol, our body tells our brain to turn off the endorphin production. The body can recognize that we have endorphins already circulating in our system so there is no need for the brain to produce any more. After years of on and off behavior, it becomes more difficult for the body to turn back on its normal endorphin production. We become more and more dependent upon using external endorphins (such as opiates and alcohol) to maintain some level of mental sanity. Without our endorphins, the simple task of waking up in the morning, showering, putting on clean clothes and going to work may become one of the most incredibly stressful moments of our life. If this is stressful, take it to the next level of needing to manage employees, pay mortgages, feed our children, discuss finances with our spouse or any other normal function we do on a daily basis. At this point, addiction has taken over, denial is in full force, and we are secretly getting loaded every day as the cycle just keeps spiraling down.

Now, if we add some type of stimulant in daily use, such as cocaine or methamphetamines, an entirely new layer of dysfunction is attained. Yes, the cocaine intoxication is intense with this overwhelming feeling of confidence and self-assuredness; however, the pleasure is short lived and replaced with shaky hands and an internal combustion that has us sweating while standing still. Believe me, this is anything but glamorous and fun. The trouble is, with our decreased endorphins from all of our opiate and alcohol use, our self-confidence is completely gone, and, for fleeting moments, it can be restored ten-fold with a line of pharmaceutical cocaine.

As cocaine or methamphetamine use increases, our body begins to become depleted of dopamine. Dopamine is one of the main neurotransmitters that sends messages between nerve endings. Without adequate amounts of dopamine in our brain, we begin to exhibit a cocaine induced psychosis. We can experience hallucinations, and commonly, extreme paranoia.

The good news is, if we don't die of an overdose, we can recover. It may take many months; however, our body will begin producing endorphins again and we will replenish our dopamine reserves. At some point we are able to manage life, show up when we are needed, and be present for the ones we love.

***

It is not my intention to tell ugly drug stories; however, now, and again, some real-life episodes need to be revealed to whoever is reading this, so they have a glimpse into the crazy life Susie, and I were going through.

During the final six months of my using, I began to experience cocaine induced psychosis. At some point I noticed I had a little pimple on my forehead just between my eyes. Most likely, had I put a dab of salicylic acid gel on it, by the next morning it would have been dried up and gone. Instead, I began to pick at it, wanting to extract the white puss. After a couple days of this, I was certain there was a nodule stuck in my forehead. I tried using tweezers to pull it out and all I got was a chunk of bloody tissue. After a week of this my wound was the size of a quarter and getting worse. Puss was beginning to form under the skin and my forehead was puffy from one side to the other. I could press down on my forehead with my finger and puss would ooze out any pore that would allow it.

One would think this would be enough to get me to seek help for my drug use. Nope, instead I went to the urgent care and made up some story about bumping my head on a dirty beam while I was crawling under our house doing some plumbing. They gave me a course of antibiotics and sent me on my way, no questions asked.

During the middle of this, I packed up my wife and children and took them to my sister's house in Arcata for two nights during Thanksgiving. What an incredibly irresponsible mess I was. I had brought enough drugs hidden with me to last a few days; however, within six hours I had taken them all. I then proceeded to lay in bed all day long Thanksgiving Day and night, complaining that my forehead was causing flu symptoms. I left Susie to look after the kids and visit with my family while I slept and sweated. I was 24 hours past my last use when I found a bottle of hydrocodone tablets in the bathroom cabinet. I immediately took them as mine, swallowed nine tablets, and within 30 minutes I was miraculously cured of my flu. I spent the rest of the afternoon and evening visiting with everyone as if nothing at all was out of the ordinary.

We packed up the next morning to drive home to Santa Cruz. By the time we got home I was once again beginning to go into withdrawals, so I volunteered to go out and get us some Chinese food for dinner. Of course, my plan was to stop by the pharmacy, unlock the doors, turn off the alarm, and use some opiates and cocaine. By time I got back with the Chinese food Susie had the children bathed and, in their pajamas, ready for bed. I had been gone over one and one-half hours and I had to tell Susie a lie about how the place was busy, and I had to wait for them to get the food ready.

These days, I am acutely aware of any physical manifestation that may preempt an emotional agenda. To clarify, if I find myself picking at acne on my forehead, I immediately need to ask myself what is going on that I need to address. Have I recently been rude to someone, was I in a conversation where I didn't listen appropriately, was I acting the know-it-all scenario? The point is, this physical action of picking at my face triggers my conscience to evaluate my recent past, critically, for any unresolved personal or emotional issues. My job then is to meditate on the situation, talk to someone if necessary, and come up with the best action to resolve the issue.

***

Reflecting back on the winter of 1996 I am amazed at how clearly I can remember the emotions that were spinning around in our home. Enough so that just meditating on it for a few minutes creates an anxious feeling in my gut.

Maybe I would come home an hour late from work, dinner would be cold, and the kids already ate. Susie would be angry and frustrated with me for not calling, and I would get upset back at her with a self-righteous lie. This would escalate to yelling with confused anger from Susie, not understanding why I was becoming so increasingly erratic, and I would argue back, digging myself deeper and deeper into my lie, trying to make her understand. All the while, our two and four year-old children were in the next room watching a show or playing with each other, feeling all of the emotions that were swirling around the home.

Unknowingly, I would walk into the house reeking of anxiety and fear, absolutely petrified of how I was going to make it through the evening as a husband and father. Susie would be waiting for me with anger and frustration from my lack of communication and rapidly decreasing level of parental responsiveness. After 30 minutes with each other we couldn't help but soak up each other's emotions, creating an ever-expanding dysfunctional mess.

In counseling school, we learned that in order to be present, emotionally, for anyone else, ever, we first need to be in touch with our own emotions. The idea is, at any point in time, we can take five seconds and recognize the emotion we are currently feeling. This process of recognizing your current emotion is called shoe-horning.

We all have the capability to do this; however, it takes practice. First of all, we need to understand that, on any given day, we will experience quite a number of different emotions. It's entirely possible that within 30 minutes we may be devastated, happy, angry, cheerful, anxious, or perhaps just plain old good. The trick is, knowing yourself well enough to be able to shoe-horn yourself and define exactly which emotion you are feeling at any given point in time.

The next step in this process is to understand the concept that emotions are transmissible. Yes, I have my emotions and you have yours; however, if I am not conscious of my own current emotions, I may inadvertently begin feeling what you are feeling.

Have you ever been sitting in a room, perhaps you are feeling relatively pleasant, then someone walks in and you all of a sudden get this horribly uncomfortable feeling? Most likely you are picking up on the other person's emotions.

As a general rule, this process helps people communicate and understand each other just a little better. In a counseling session, shoe-horning yourself and then feeling the emotions of the individual sitting across from you may provide the link to real help.

Before you meet with your client, you shoe-horn yourself and get a good reading on your current emotion. Now, when the client walks in and sits down, you again continue to shoe-horn yourself to feel if your emotions are changing.

As they change, define them for yourself. Most likely, these new feelings are the emotions that your client just brought into the room. As you may have guessed, drug addicts and alcoholics in counseling are not always the most forthcoming with true information. Ideally, a seasoned counselor, with a good understanding of their own emotions, will recognize when an individual is talking about one topic; however, their emotions are telling another story.

The reason I am discussing all of this is because it made such a huge impact on my recovery lifestyle. The concept of being present and still long enough to actually feel my own emotions, and then understand what the person next to me might be feeling, was far more than I had hoped to ever understand. Furthermore, this concept brought home hours of communication for Susie and I, taking the time to discuss our emotions and recognize them within each other.

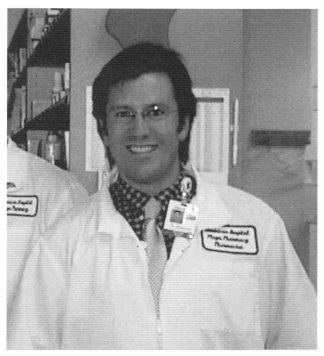

Steve as a young pharmacist just starting at Dominican, 1998.

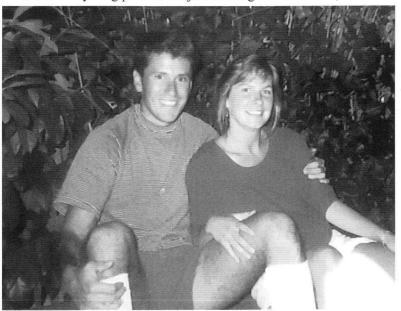

Steve and Susie, summer of '88.

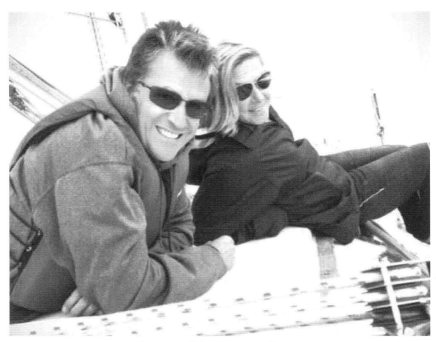

Steve and Susie out sailing.

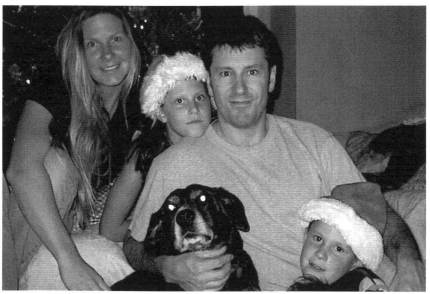

Christmas as a young, and recovering, family.

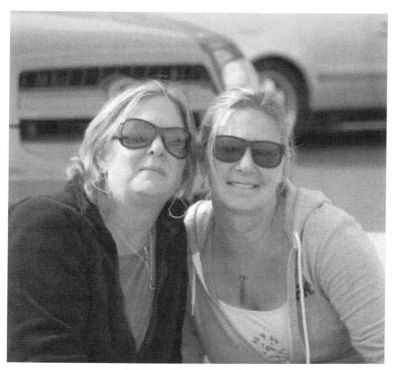

Susie and her sister Janet.

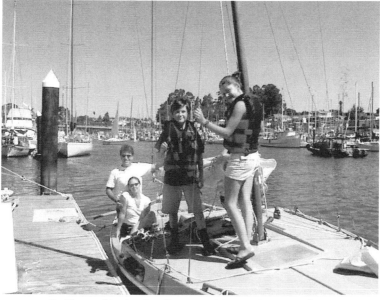

Sailing with the family out of Santa Cruz Harbor.

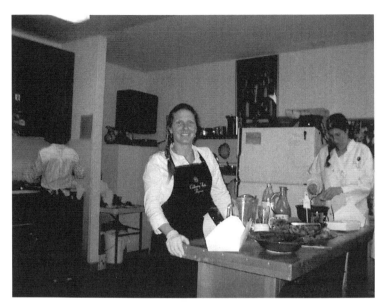

Susie in class at Culinary School.

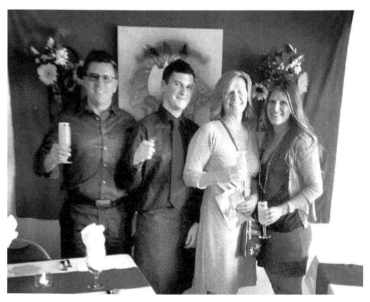

Cooper, graduation day at Culinary School.

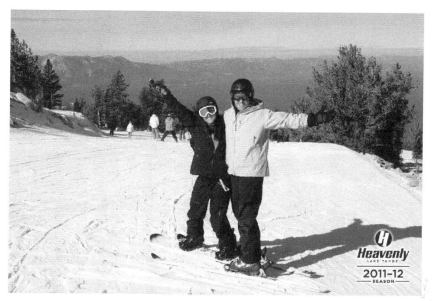

Many years riding the runs of Heavenly Valley with Kendyl.

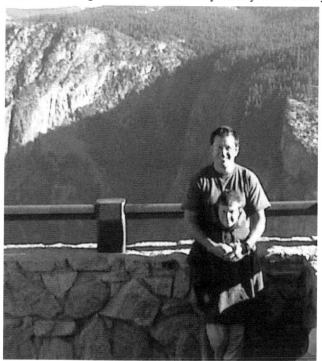

One of the early trips to Yosemite with Cooper.

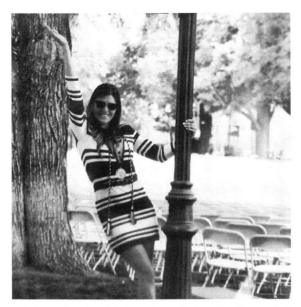

Kendyl graduating University of Nevada, Reno, 2013.

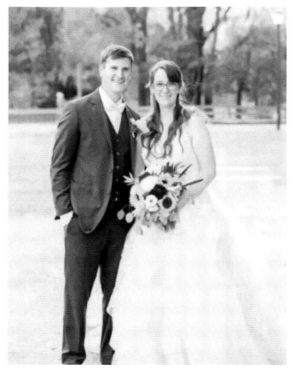

Cooper and Deanna, 10-1-2021

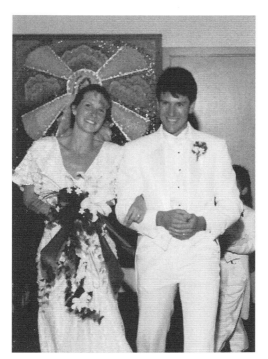

Susie and Steve 7-7-1990

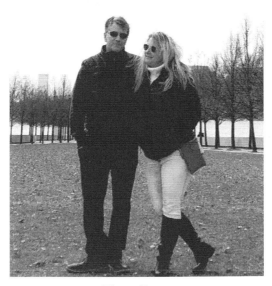

These Days

19

Practicing Again

Just as I was finishing up the two semester Certification Program for Addiction Counseling (CPAC), I read in the newspaper there was an opening for a pharmacist at Dominican Hospital. It had been just over 15 months since I had last stepped into a pharmacy. Honestly, over the previous year, I really did not know if I would ever be ready to work as a practicing pharmacist again. After some long discussions with Susie, my therapist, and my health professional drug addict group, we agreed it would be a good idea for me to update my resume and apply for the position.

The day came for my interview and I walked in the front doors of Dominican Hospital. Interestingly, I felt oddly at ease sitting in the lobby of the hospital waiting for the pharmacy manager to come and greet me. There was a feeling like I had come back home.

Throughout the past seven years, as well as a few years in college, I had become very familiar with the sights, sounds, and smells of a hospital. This is a very comforting feeling, coming back to an incredibly familiar environment, especially since I had completely forgotten the feelings it gave me.

As I sat down for the interview with the director of the pharmacy department, as well as the pharmacy manager, I was able to check my emotions and realize I was actually feeling incredibly relaxed. Very little feeling of anxiety and definitely not nervous. Over the years I have realized that if all I have is the truth in my heart, brain and tongue, the rest of my body will follow with pleasant relaxation.

After our introductions and pleasantries, and before either of them had a moment to ask any specific questions, I asked if it would be appropriate for me to share my history with them. In my mind, the only way I was going to be able to come back and work in a pharmacy is if, from the very first moment, I was truthful and honest about all things. I shared with them how I had turned myself in for stealing and using drugs. As well, I discussed the inpatient recovery program I attended, therapy, and counseling school. After my15-minute story, they both thanked me for my candor and appreciated my direct honesty. We talked about pharmacy for another 20 minutes and the next day they called me and offered me the job.

Remember how I was talking about miracles a few pages back, well, here's another one. I graduated from the Bethany College CPAC program in June of 1997, and then started practicing pharmacy again at Dominican Hospital the very next month.

Santa Cruz is quite a small town. The pharmacy had, at that time, maybe eight pharmacists and 10 technicians working various shifts. I was acutely aware, even before I walked through the main pharmacy door for my first shift, that each and every one of them knew I had gone to a drug and alcohol treatment program and had been out of work for 15 months. It was my current goal to walk into work, be prepared to learn, and not concern myself with anyone else's opinion of what I had gone through.

As I had learned in therapy, one of my main defects was an incredibly overrated concern about what other people thought of me. I was a people pleaser and continually drove satisfaction out of praise from other individuals. Through working the 12-steps, as well as lengthy discussions in therapy, I came to understand that my satisfaction in my actions comes from my inner self as well as my higher power. Never will the praise of others be enough to satisfy an addict's need for gratification. Only when I accept that I am solely responsible for my actions am I able to be present with others who have differing or misguided opinions of who I am or what I have done.

As I have learned, the way to gain the trust of your colleagues is to show up early, do more than is expected, ask for help when necessary and take notes so you do not need to ask a second time, never gossip, always be polite, answer the phone on the first ring, if you step in the problem it's yours, don't be a know-it-all, know your boundaries, and I'll say it one more time, show up early. After three or four weeks at the hospital I had been given the opportunity to work shifts with just about everyone on staff. Of course, everyone has their own personality; however, I felt welcome.

***

Have you ever heard the phrase, "waiting for the next shoe to drop"? Well, three months into my new job, and 18 months into recovery, the next shoe dropped. Susie met me at the door when I got home from work. The look on her face was one of fear. She had received a large manila envelope via certified mail that afternoon. It was addressed to me and was from the California State Board of Pharmacy.

We opened the envelope and began to read our way through the pages. The State of California was filing a lawsuit against me, with the goal of revoking my pharmacist license. We both were devastated. How could this be? I had turned myself in, done everything exactly as it had been laid out in front of me, and now this. Come to find out, even though I had turned myself in, I had still been negligent in my practice of pharmacy and the State Board of Pharmacy was prepared to administer disciplinary action.

After reading the entire legal document, spelling out exactly which laws I had broken in exquisite detail, I was certain that I did not deserve to practice pharmacy ever again. This was it, both Susie and I were preparing ourselves for what would happen to us. Fortunately, I had a program in place to help manage my big decisions so I wouldn't make

122

them all on my own. Therapy, AA meetings, and importantly, the health care professional therapy group I went to each week.

The next meeting I had with the group, which came around quickly being that we had them every week, I asked for some time to discuss my legal situation. Walking through the process, I shared how the state had spelled out all of my wrong doings and dishonest pharmacy practices as well as how they felt it necessary to revoke my license and disallow me from every practicing pharmacy again. In their great wisdom, the group looked at me and asked me if this person they are describing is the same person sitting in the room with them tonight. I assured them that absolutely not, the person sitting in the room with them tonight is honest, truthful, willing, and clinically appropriate in all matters.

One by one, they all assured me that today I am not the same person who had committed the negligent practice the legal documents are referring to. Yes, it was me; however, today I am a changed individual. I am a qualified and competent pharmacist working in a professional and appropriate capacity. After much more discussion, they assured me that my job, here and now, is to hire a lawyer and let them work it out with the California State Board of Pharmacy.

Within a couple weeks, Susie and I were sitting in a lawyer's office discussing our case. After what seemed a lifetime of months, another certified letter came in the mail. This was our official settlement with the State of California. My license was now revoked for 12 months, to be followed with five years probation, and I was required to participate in the pharmacist recovery program. Fortunately, from day one I had been participating in the pharmacist recovery program and had already completed 15 months of not practicing pharmacy. The state appreciated my efforts toward recovery as well as my complete and full participation in all required meetings, so they gave me time served on all accounts. At this time, I just needed to complete an additional three years of probation and my license would be free and clear.

Now and again, I like to refer back to the miracles that have been happening in my life. One of the stipulations of my probation was that I was not allowed to be the only pharmacist in the pharmacy at any point in time. This would be a difficult stipulation to satisfy at many institutions or pharmacies; however, my current job was already structured so just about every shift available had two pharmacists on duty. The miracle is, I had already been placed in a pharmacist position that met all of the stipulations of my probation with regards to practicing pharmacy on a daily basis.

Over the next few years, the recovery process became second nature. Meetings with the health professional group and therapy just became part of who I was and what I did. The therapy portion actually became quite satisfying. I remember thinking that, in my opinion, everyone should have the opportunity to attend three or four years of therapy in order to better understand who they are and where their thoughts and actions came from.

Sometime after four years of probation in the pharmacist's recovery program I got an idea that I might like to petition the board of pharmacy for early termination. After doing my research I completed the application for early termination and received approval to sit before the pharmacy board members at one of the quarterly meetings. I had submitted a packet with letters of recommendation from physicians, pharmacists, and hospital managers as well as my complete participation in the state mandated pharmacist recovery program.

It just so happened that this particular meeting was taking place in San Diego, so I scheduled a flight and made plans to stay with my nephew Dave and his new wife Jen (both pharmacists) at their home just a few miles away from the meeting site. I remember feeling both confident and butterfly nervous as I was called up to the front of the room to sit in front of the 10 or so board members. They were all sitting behind a row of tables at the front end of a hotel conference hall, and I was asked to sit in a chair, about 15 feet in front of them. From my chair I had a clear vision of the entire group.

After about five minutes of answering their questions, I was beginning to realize I was a little bit of an anomaly. It was beginning to become clear to me that pharmacists usually don't complete the entire recovery program, or if they do, it's only after a relapse of some kind and a start over. The feeling in the room quickly changed from an inquisition to more of an inquisitive question and answer session. These board members wanted to know how I had done it when so many others failed. Within a short couple weeks, I had received yet another certified letter from the California State Board of Pharmacy. This time it was the board stating they were releasing me from probation six months early based upon my exemplary performance in the pharmacist recovery program and my full integration back into pharmacy practice.

After many years of practice, in December of 2018 I had the honor of posting an article about recovery in the State Board of Pharmacy quarterly newsletter for the entire 40,000 licensed California pharmacists to read.

> *Every even year in October, since 1987, I have had the privilege of renewing my pharmacist license with the California State Board of Pharmacy. I say privilege because that is exactly what it is. If I honor a certain code of conduct, maintain my practice, complete the requisite number of continuing education hours, and send them a check, they will do me the honor of renewing my license for another two years.*

> *Just the other day I completed my continuing education for this licensing cycle and sent off my check. After about two weeks I noticed my check had been cashed; however, I had not yet received my license in the mail. Fortunately, the California State Board of Pharmacy has an excellent public website where anyone can type in the name of a pharmacist and obtain the current license status of that individual. I proceeded to do just that and found that my license was clear until October of 2020.*

LICENSE STATUS: CLEAR ⓘ **EXPIRATION DATE:** OCTOBER 31, 2020
SECONDARY STATUS: PROBATION TERMINATED/COMPLETED ⓘ

This picture from the state website is public knowledge, available for anyone who searches, so I have absolutely no problem posting it here. What caught my eye was the term SECONDARY STATUS. The state must have reconfigured their site to include the secondary status; I do not recall this being listed over the years when I have checked my license in the past. This is an excellent reminder to me of how far I have come.

One Sunday morning, in the Spring of 1996, I phoned the owner of the store that I was working at and informed him of my substance abuse addiction. I had reached the level of incomprehensible demoralization; my family life, spiritual connection and health were all rapidly deteriorating. On the phone I told my former boss I was prepared for whatever action he felt was appropriate.

In his amazing wisdom and kindness, he said, "Steve, we're going to get you some help." I met him an hour later and we were on the phone to the state board of pharmacies Pharmacist Recovery Program hotline. The next day I was enrolled in a 28-day inpatient treatment program, learning the tools of recovery.

Although there were no criminal charges filed, I did make a statement to the board of pharmacy, describing specifically any controlled substances I had taken from the store. For my negligent actions, the state board of pharmacy placed my license on five years' probation. After four and one-half years I appealed, and my license was released from probation.

Now, 23 uninterrupted years later, I am still alcohol and substance free. My family life is lovely, I am spiritually connected, and I have been practicing in the same outpatient pharmacy for 21 years.

Current studies show that up to 15% of nurses, doctors and pharmacists will misuse or abuse controlled substances, without

126

a prescription, during their career. Another recent study shows that up to 46% of all pharmacists have used a controlled substance at some point without a prescription.

We think we can control it...until we can't.

"Institutional, local, and statewide impaired-physician programs are now available for the active treatment and rehabilitation of impaired healthcare professionals. Many of these programs are also designed to assist the clinician with reentry into clinical practice. Rarely is punitive action taken when the healthcare provider undergoes successful treatment and ongoing follow-up management. Overall recovery rates for impaired healthcare professionals seem to be higher compared with other groups, particularly with intensive inpatient management and subsequent follow-up care."

The California Pharmacists Recovery Program is an excellent resource. As stated on the program's web page, "Through this program, the chemically dependent or mentally troubled pharmacist is provided with the hope and assistance required for a successful recovery."

20

Spirit World

When I think of Dad, practical and organized come to mind. Go to school, get a job, and never go without some kind of medical insurance. Stay in constant contact with your debtors to maintain good credit, return phone calls, always follow through and do what you said you are going to do and never strike your children. Dad was a good man.

Dad lived on his own for quite a few years after Mom passed away. Having eight children and numerous grandchildren he always had company; however, he lived alone. Amongst other visits, I would stop by once weekly to help him with his weekly pill box. He didn't take much, some blood pressure and cholesterol medication and maybe a little pain medication now and again.

After a few years he began missing a day of medication now and again. No big deal, it was just surprising, because Dad was usually not the forgetful type. Then, one afternoon I stopped by and most of the pill box was still full of the previous week. A couple of the pills were gone, but there was no pattern to be seen. I asked Dad what was going on and he said he was irritated and agitated and didn't know why he had to take all these pills.

Soon after that visit we had a doctor's appointment where Dad tried to discuss how he felt. The doctor gave Dad and anti-depressant medication to help him with his agitation and anxiety. As we know, these medications work well; however, they need to be taken on a regular basis and also may make an individual feel a little out-of-sorts for the first week or two of therapy. Dad took it for a couple days, didn't like how it made him feel, and wouldn't take it again.

This cycle went around and around for six or eight months. Dad was becoming acutely disoriented, rapidly confused and increasingly agitated. Eventually my brothers, sisters and I began taking turns staying over at his house. I wish I could say I was a completely compassionate son and was totally understanding of his situation. I found myself becoming frustrated and angry with Dad for getting so agitated over the littlest of things.

What we didn't know at the time is that Dad would be diagnosed, two weeks before he passed away, with lung cancer, from his work with asbestos on airplanes back in the 40's. The cancer had spread to his brain and was affecting his entire thought process.

We were able to do a reasonable renovation on a portion of our garage and create a studio for Dad to move into. He was reluctant because the move was conditional upon Dad giving up his car. He felt very dependent upon his vehicle and was increasingly unsure of how he would get around without it. After plenty of reassurance, he agreed to donate his car to his granddaughter and come live in our little cottage. I was amazed at how calm and relaxed Dad would become when Susie would sit and listen to his stories for hours at a time.

We could see the back door to the cottage from our upstairs bedroom window. Early after Dad moved in, Susie noticed the porch light from the cottage go on at about four in the morning. Dad was dressed and heading outside. Susie promptly got up and went down to meet Dad outside. She pleasantly asked him if everything was alright and he, matter of fact, stated that it was time to get up and milk the cows. Susie then proceeded to invite Dad in for coffee and oatmeal, letting him know that he should most likely eat a little breakfast first. After an hour sitting around the dining room table Dad pleasantly got up and up and went back down to his cottage to rest.

Having Dad around, on the property, was wonderful for our kids. Even though Dad was becoming increasingly more confused, he was still present with our children with a gentle soul and kind heart. Dad passed away two months after he moved in with us. It was quick and the Hospice team was here to help all of us (brothers, sisters, in-laws, grandkids etc.) deal with the process.

Remembering when Mom passed, I could feel her presence for months to come, as if she had unfinished business here on this earthly space. This was not the case when Dad passed. Both Susie and I felt this rush of wind and then poof, he was absolutely gone. I can only imagine how elated he was to be with his lovely wife once again in heaven. As well, his mother who died when he was just a toddler and all of the other adults from his young life growing up on Lake McDonald in Glacier Park and the farm in Wisconsin.

***

As I just described, Dad's presence was gone immediately; however, Mom's hung around for quite a while. While I was still working at Medical Clinic Pharmacy in Santa Cruz, just prior to becoming sober, my schedule involved me showing up at the midtown pharmacy just before 8am. After helping to get the store opened and moving, I would head cross town to the west-side pharmacy where I would open the store at 9am and work until close at 6pm. The main roads were always a bit crowded, so I enjoyed taking some side streets, through the neighborhoods, working my way through downtown, past the high school and up to the west-side pharmacy.

This one particular morning, I came to a stop sign at a four way stop that would lead down the hill and through town. When I came to a stop in my Scout, I noticed there was a cat lying in the intersection. Upon quick further inspection, I could see that the back half of the cat had been run over and was basically flat on the road. With what little life it had left, the cat was trying to push up with his two front legs to pull himself up.

Wright or wrong, I made a decision in that split second that I could not let that cat suffer one more moment. I pulled from the stop sign and with my large 4X4 tires, drove right over the top of him to instantly relieve his misery.

At that moment, out of the corner of my eye, I see a young woman sitting behind the driver's seat of a small sedan at the stop sign to my left. To this day I can still see the look of horror over her face being the only human witness to the mayhem just committed in front of her.

As I described earlier, at this point, my life was falling apart due to an ever-increasing need for opiates, cocaine and a continually increasing stream of lies. This split-second decision to run over the mutilated cat followed by the look of horror from the young lady witness, I am sure, was a jolt from my higher power to ask for help.

Within seconds of pulling away from the intersection I could physically feel large feathery wings reaching around my entire body and holding me with the words, "It's going to be alright" coming into my head. This was my guardian angel, my past mother. Over the next four or five months, or however long it took until that moment where I called for help, she was with me. I could feel her presence, watching me, continually trying to guide me.

There was a moment about six months after I became sober. I was sitting in the kitchen, and I can't remember what it was that we were discussing or specifically doing; however, it was crystal clear, in that moment, that my guardian angel, my mother, knew I was going to be safe, and she left.

21

Family Life in Recovery

Wonder Years

For quite some time now I've referred to the time between when the kids started elementary school and when they graduate high school as the wonder years. For me, this is the age of wonder. Kids wonder what life will be like when they get older. Life is slowly revealed to them, and, as they grow, more ideas come into place, increasing the ability to wonder what tomorrow will bring. As well, parents continually wonder if they are doing the right thing with their kids. As parents, we take what we have learned, combine it with what our partner has learned, discuss it, try to throw out the bad and implement the good, and wonder if it is all going to work.

Early on, everything felt so incredibly centered around home. We are a core group, mom, dad and two kids, eating together, traveling as a group, celebrating all of our holidays as a unit, and feeling each other's emotions all the time. The children grow and naturally the core group seems to fade. We experience times through the early teens where it feels like the core will come close to being ripped apart; however, it doesn't. Then again, later, toward the end of the teens the core once again tightens back up a little, in a different way.

For us it's maybe about a 10-year time span that starts sometimes around six years old. I understand every family experiences this to some degree or another, perhaps with more children or maybe with only one child and for fewer years. Our experience is not unique; however, it also may be considered the most incredibly unique experience our family has ever had.

To be clear, this is my version of the wonder years. My experience, when taking time to meditate back on those incredibly special years, may be seen differently than my wife or two children. The external description of experiences may be seen differently when viewing them through my memory as opposed to the recollection of the rest of our core family; however, the emotions we all experienced throughout the time were palpable and resonate through time.

If you haven't noticed by now, I am big on emotions. Feeling, expressing, discussing, and living our true and authentic self is how we integrate ourselves into the lives of those around us. We learn how what we say may create an emotional response in someone we love. In times of great happiness, our thoughtful words of excitement may precipitate extreme joy and happiness in those close to us. As well, when we are feeling anger and emotional pain our outpouring of harsh words may create an intense hurtful response in our close family members. Certainly, this is not new news to anyone who has grown up in a family. As a close family, we open up our hearts with each other, and sometimes we intentionally hurt each other. The beauty is, we are each other's family, we communicate, we forgive, and we move on.

Continuing my common theme of miracles happening in daily life, this particular miracle is a little broader reaching, like a fishing net cast out over my life. I am referring to the extension of my sobriety, which brought truth and authenticity into my being and allowed me to be present, on a daily basis, for my family. I'm thinking the wonder years, in our house, began just about the same time I was hired at Dominican Hospital Pharmacy, in the summer of 1997. Kendyl turned six years old and started 1st grade that fall.

My life had become so incredibly simple. Wake up in the morning and have coffee with Susie, help get the kids ready for school, go to work and do my job, come home and be present with my family, help the kids get ready for bed, and hang out with my wife. My personal world had ceased spinning and was no longer causing a crisis in anyone's life. Now that I was working again, Susie was able to cut back on her work at the medical clinic and be present with the children after school.

As a family, we have many layers to unfold, such as what we do, how we feel, our interactions with each other and the role we play in the group. This discussion alone could get deep and go on for pages; however, that is not my intent. We all have our own story about this time in our life, and I don't want to take anyone else's story away from them. The layer that I will attempt to unfold is how, when one person stops spinning, another may pick it up and start spinning.

For years Susie had been holding the house together through my chaos. After I came home from the treatment facility, she continued to hold the house together by stepping up and getting a full-time job to supplement our house income so we could continue to live in our home. When I went back to work, Susie was then able to come back home and step back into her stay-at-home mom position again; however, this time it was different. This time, there was no crisis to manage, just life. This was different than before. Through our ever-expanding ability to communicate, and time, Susie was able to let go of the crisis management mode and fulfill her immediate future with the pleasures of being present for our children both before and after school.

It's difficult to discern how having a drug addict or alcoholic creating chaos in a home will affect young children as they grow up. Fortunately, our children were only exposed to the turmoil for a few of their young years; however, it was absolutely real in our house, and they were part of it. Both Susie and I had sought help for ourselves as well as our relationship. With this in mind, whenever we had concerns for our children's well-being, we knew there was help and how to get it.

***

With life not spinning out of control anymore, our family began to develop its groove. For the next four or five years we participated in a lovely version of family dynamics. Dad was still at the center of our larger family and our house became a gathering place for holidays and Saturday BBQ's. Susie, bless her soul, would help orchestrate the house so everyone always felt comfortable and at home. It seemed as though on any given weekend we were always having either a sleepover with a handful of cousins or some sort of family food festival where everyone would gather throughout the house and yard.

From our perspective, this is what life was meant to be. Yes, our house was an old Victorian farmhouse that had yet to be renovated; however, we had room for family to relax, extra room for kids to play, and love. It was quite common to have a bonfire in the pit out back and we would all sit around well into the dark hours roasting marshmallows, telling stories, and watching the kids play. The excitement of the kids playing always led to some sort of play or dance production. Someone would orchestrate the players, direct the others in a collaboration, and before long a wild and noisy production would be working its way across our little deck.

As happens over time, things change. Susie's sister, sadly, moved with her husband and two children to St. George, Utah. We had grown to know her children quite well in the few short years we had with them; however, now that they were over 13 hours' drive away, we would see them maybe once every two years or so. Around the same time, my brothers children moved up north with their mother. Fortunately, we were able to see them a little now and again; however, it was never like it was for those few short years. To top it all off, Dad passed away.

Our house had been a gathering place for brothers and sisters and Dad for a few special years. I know big families always promise to keep getting together the same way they did when their parents were alive. Maybe some do. In our family, this was about the time that all of our kids were beginning to get older. We all develop our own family dynamic and create our own gatherings with our own core family at the center. Some of my siblings we see and participate with in life on a relatively regular basis, others we see one or two times per year. Fortunately, our young children were able to have the experience of big family gatherings and many close cousins for a few amazing years.

***

Every summer the Boardwalk has a concert series. Fun music, bands that have, well, maybe just can't fill a stadium anymore. We would take the kids to the beach on Friday evening during the summer and listen to the music for an hour or so. One evening rolls clearly in my mind. Middle of summer and at 6:30 pm the sun is still shining, and shorts and t-shirts are still just fine. The fog hasn't quite rolled in yet and the sounds of the roller coaster and bumper cars are ringing through the air. Susie, Cooper, and I laid out our beach blanket and bag of snacks and drinks for the show.

The band America is performing. I couldn't believe America was actually playing here, at the Boardwalk, for free. This is one of the bands I grew up with in the early 70's. I knew the words to each and every song they played. We were off in the distance, so we had room to play in the sand, stand up, dance, and move around without getting in the way of the concert goers who were sitting and watching the show. Dancing with Kendyl, who was maybe seven years old at the time, I remember tossing her up into the sky, seeing her float effortlessly with her blond hair hanging in the sun, and then catching her as we swing with the groove of the music. Susie and Cooper swing dancing, with Susie giving Cooper a picturesque twirl under her arm, smiles from ear to ear.

***

When I was a kid in the middle of my wonder years, beginning the summer after 2nd grade, Mom and Dad took us camping in Yosemite every year for summer vacation. These were amazing two week long adventure trips. Mom and Dad would set up camp in the Curry Village housekeeping tent cabins and we would follow with lovely days and nights of hiking, roasting marshmallows, bike riding and adventures. These were family trips where usually it was just me and Mom and Dad for the entire time; however, brothers and sisters and their kids would all come for three or four nights at different times throughout the weeks.

These trips made a big impact on my life as a child. When I have an incredibly stressful time in my work life, phones ringing and patients lining up outside the pharmacy, I can draw upon the feeling of the warm sun on my face as I stand on the sandy beach of the Merced River, just down from our tent cabin, throwing the football back and forth with my Dad. This memory grounds me. As a parent, I wanted to be able to share that emotional place with my kids.

As it turned out, Susie and I never really migrated toward camping. Yes, we are very adventurous in our own way; however, as a family, camping never really took on. Fortunately, I still had the opportunity to share Yosemite with both of our children in an offbeat way.

First off, when Susie and I were dating and we were both living in Santa Cruz, we had the opportunity to go camping in Yosemite. My oldest brother was one of the amazing few individuals who had both the talent and the gumption to run off the top of Glacier Point strapped into a hang glider. On one of his first summers doing this, many of our family traveled to Yosemite, set up camp at Bridal Veil Falls campground on the Glacier Point highway, and cheered on when he landed in the meadows on the Yosemite Valley floor. Not only was I excited to take Susie to Yosemite and go camping with her, but it was also exciting having her hang out with our family around the campfire.

My brother John kept up his flying off Glacier Point for quite a few years. When Cooper was about eight or 9, we started a tradition of driving up to Yosemite to camp for a couple nights and drive for John. He needed someone to drive his car back down from the top of Glacier Point to the meadow down below. Usually this involved two days of flying, so on one of the days we would stay up top until take off, so we could watch John run down the long stretch with his glider and take off into the sky. The next day we would drop off John and then drive down to the valley. We would arrive just in time to watch him land on the big meadow. It takes about 60 minutes to do the drive, and only about 20 minutes for the flight.

The first two years we did this involved us just parking alongside the road and walking about a half mile and finding someplace to camp. Maybe not the most legal way of Yosemite camping; however, quite fun, and very exciting for both me and Cooper. I remember the first night doing this with John and Cooper. It was after 9pm that we met up with John in Yosemite. We parked and walked for about 30 minutes in the dark on a trail, looking for someplace to lay down our sleeping bags. We got back to our truck the next morning to find our SUV was gone. It had been towed. We had left an ice chest in the back of it and the rangers will tow any vehicle with visible food storage in order to prevent bear damage. Lesson learned.

The third trip to Yosemite with Cooper we decided to extend the adventure and make it a father and son camping trip. We got to Yosemite a few days before the hang glider crew so we could do some river swimming and trail hiking. Cooper, with his 10-year-old legs, hiked 10 miles with me out of Tuolumne Meadows to a waterfall and back. The trail was lovely; however, the feeling of spending time like this on the trail with my son was amazing.

The trips I had to Yosemite with Kendyl were unique, unlike anything I ever expected to do as a parent. Throughout Kendyl's three years in middle school, she played the clarinet in the school band. The band was great, cohesive, and very talented. Her band leader, Mr. Fred, had an established event once a year to perform a concert for the Yosemite Valley school district. Parents would be asked to chaperone, maybe about one parent for every five or seven kids or so, and we would all ride up to Yosemite in two big, chartered buses. The kids would help set up right when we got there and perform a short concert for the school kids. Then, later on that evening, they would perform a more formal show for all of the local parents and families of the Yosemite Valley school kids. They would host a nice spaghetti feed and then, we would lay out our sleeping pads and sleeping bags in the school hallway for the long night of middle school talking and or maybe some sleeping.

In-between setting up, performing, eating, and sleeping we had some free time to go out and do a little bit of adventuring. Even though I was there as Kendyl's dad, and she was looking for an increasing amount of freedom, I could tell that she still really appreciated having me close by. We have this one lovely photo of Kendyl snuggling up next to me on a carved log bench near the lower Yosemite falls bridge, absolutely priceless.

Three years in a row I had the opportunity to participate in this wonderful event. Each year I could see Kendyl become a little more independent, as well as an ever-improving clarinet player. The first year we went I was able to sit next to her on the bus. By the third year, I was fortunate to be on the same bus as she was. I am pretty sure she knew I was always keeping an eye out for her, and she knew she could find me at a moment's notice if she ever needed me right away.

***

Through our children's early teens our house was a common hangout place for many of their friends. We created what we thought was an environment conducive to happy engagement with friends. Sleep-overs were common, late night summer swimming parties in our above ground pool were exciting, fantastic Saturday and Sunday morning breakfasts complete with cinnamon fluff French toast were always greeted with smiles and communication was valued at its highest level.

The wonder years bring to mind a sense of nostalgia. As I sit here, I remember one memory after another, all of which would create an interesting timeline of events; however, once again, this story is much more about emotions than events. Many of the stories are not necessarily mine to tell, they are centered around Cooper and Kendyl and the experiences they shared. Someday I look forward to hearing and reading their version of the wonder years. Until then, I'll enjoy my memories.

When I was growing up in Ben Lomond, we had this little wooden art piece hanging in the kitchen that stated, "Our house is clean enough to be healthy and dirty enough to be happy". We all happily lived in our space, got in each other's way on a regular basis, and let each other have their own time whenever they needed it.

Culinary Institute

Susie has always been amazing in the kitchen. I remember when we lived in Mt. Shasta in our first house on Lassen Lane, Susie would make this delicious filet of sole under paper. She would serve it, somehow under this balloon type parchment paper, that she would pop open at the table and reveal this lovely slice of fish with vegetables.

For years, way before its time, Susie understood the importance of cooking with organic, fresh whole foods. Unfortunately, the kids and I weren't quite there yet and didn't fully understand the passion she felt for creating both delicious and incredibly healthy and nutritious meals. Fortunately for us, our inability to see her vision did not slow her down in her desire to learn and grow gastronomically as well as continue to feed us with healthy food choices.

During the kid's 6th and 8th grade years, Susie went back to school for six months and became a Certified Whole Food Chef at the Bauman College Culinary School. This is absolutely no easy task. She attended a local culinary academy full time for six months, learning everything necessary to plan and prepare incredible whole food meals as well as manage and run a professional kitchen. All these years later, I'm still not certain if Susie had plans of working professionally as a chef; however, I am certain she wanted to be the most prepared so she could feed her family the healthiest and most nutritious delicious meals ever consumed.

As a husband watching, I saw the excitement and dreams of a young adult come true. The effort and labor Susie would undertake each week in order to excel at the current lesson plan was inspiring. The binders of recipes and techniques, all practiced and perfected. In addition, each and every day we all came to look forward to the leftovers she would bring home from school for us to sample.

For Susie's graduation, the whole chef class prepared a lovely meal for the families of the students. We all sat together in a beautifully decorated main school classroom. The culinary students would announce the meal and then serve it to us. As a husband and father, seeing Susie graduate as a certified Chef was one of the proudest moments I have experienced. As well, I know Susie was feeling similar emotions, sharing her classroom where she had spent the last six months, with her husband and children.

At the time, I am not certain the kids fully appreciated the effort Susie put into her education; however, over time I am certain they have come to fully understand all that she went through. Over the past 20 years Susie has helped me understand how food can be just as important as medicine in treating a human's body. She introduced the term SOUL food to me which stands for seasonal, organic, unprocessed, and local. We do our best to apply the SOUL food plan to all of our food shopping endeavors.

***

Interestingly, more than 10 years later, we are working with Cooper, discussing career alternatives. At the time, Cooper had been graduated from high school for about a year and was working at a local dog grooming and boarding facility. He enjoyed his work, or should I say, he enjoyed the animals he worked with. We had discussed all of the regular alternatives, such as college, trade school, military, and any other mechanism for working your way into our current world. Although Cooper was very open to all alternatives, nothing we talked about or discussed seemed to have any staying power. The one thing for certain is that he realized he didn't really want to be the guy who picked up dog poop for the rest of his working career.

At some point, the discussion of cooking came up. Susie shared her story with Cooper, about why she decided to go to Bauman College and what it taught her. This resonated with Cooper. He felt a connection to the holistic and healing nature of food and had an idea he would like to pursue this as a career. Fortunately, Bauman, at the time, had three separate campuses. One campus was in Boulder, CO, one was in Berkeley, and the other was in Santa Cruz, just two miles from our house.

Cooper enrolled in the 6-month program and began his course. To his surprise, he was the youngest student by over 10 years. Each class has 12 students that are accepted for the si month program. Students would come in from all over the country, including seasoned chef's ready to learn new skills and other adults remaking their careers. Cooper was the only student who had never worked in a kitchen. The other students accepted him as their colleague and by the time graduation came around Cooper had learned what it takes to work as a chef in this world, time, and work!

The graduation ceremony hadn't changed since Susie had graduated years earlier. The difference was, this time Susie was sitting at the table with me and Kendyl being served the incredible meals that the culinary class had prepared. Lovingly, Cooper was assigned the task by the class of announcing each meal just prior to it being served. Similar to when Susie had graduated, I was filled with such heightened emotion that it was difficult for me to speak a word without my voice cracking.

From 2003-2015 I had a part time job working a weekend shift and being the weekend on-call pharmacist for Sutter Maternity and Surgery Center in Santa Cruz. Regularly, on the weekends, either Kendyl or Cooper would come with me when I would go in to do my weekend rounds to check orders and stock. The highlight of these weekend trips was a visit to the Sutter Café where they could order whatever they like for lunch. Over the years, the cooks and other workers in the kitchen got to know Cooper and Kendyl and would say hi in a friendly way.

When Cooper was done with his culinary school, thinking about where he would apply for employment, Sutter Café was the first place that came to mind. My part was to introduce him to the current hiring manager, he did all the rest. Even though Cooper had never worked in a kitchen prior

142

to this position, they felt his commitment to completing the 6-month culinary program, as well as his glowing personal review from the dog boarding business, gave him great promise.

Cooper was hired initially as a part-time dishwasher. After two months of showing up early for his shift every time, doing a great job, and being open for learning more, they moved him into the kitchen to begin training on the cold-side as well as the order intake and cash register. Now, more than 10 years later, Cooper is one of the primary cooks at Sutter Cafe, working full time and teaching the new employees how things work.

Like I discussed earlier, the best way to create your value at your new job is to show up early, do more than is expected, ask for help when necessary and take notes so you do not need to ask a second time, never gossip, always be polite, answer the phone on the first ring, if you step in the problem it's yours, don't be a know-it-all, know your boundaries, and I'll say it one more time, show up early.

Sailing

Early on, one of the summers that we went to Utah, we left the kids with Gramma and Grandpa while Susie, and I came back early for a few days of our own in Santa Cruz. Amongst other things, we had planned for a two day sailing course out of our local harbor. Living so close to the ocean, it had been one of our dreams to learn how to sail, and, possibly, have a boat in the harbor.

We absolutely loved the class. It was just Susie and I along with the instructor on this 27-foot Santa Cruz sailboat. After learning the basics of how to sail, the instructor turned the boat over to Susie and me to run. We had a blast sailing out past the wharf, up the coast a little way, down toward Capitola, and back up toward the harbor. Along with the great teamwork we had, we also just really enjoyed the feeling of being on the ocean, floating with the waves, and watching the coastline of Santa Cruz.

That was it, we were set, we needed to get a boat.

Here's how things work in our life. Susie and I decide something, and then it happens. We have learned that we really need to be careful when it comes to this portion of our life. We both have the ability to quickly sway the other in a decision, and we are now, after many years, both very aware of this process. So, when it comes to a point where we are both on board with something happening, we have the ability to make it happen absolutely right away.

Such an incredible feeling of excitement. We had purchased a boat that had been born in the same year that I had, 1963. It was a super stable 20-foot sailboat; a Cal-20. Of course, we had given it an incredible once-over in our yard, and then after some arrangements, we had it lowered into the Santa Cruz Harbor with the yacht club's hoist. We didn't have a slip in the harbor yet; however, we wanted to give it a try, so we signed up for a temporary one-week rental slot.

Now, it was just Susie, Kendyl, Cooper, and me, ready to head out into the ocean on our own. Really, I don't think we went very far. Maybe out around the wharf, in toward the Dream Inn and then back out and around to the harbor entrance. It didn't really matter that we were only sailing for maybe one or two hours. We were all four sailing our own boat on the Monterey Bay looking back over the coastline of Santa Cruz and the Boardwalk. This was beautiful, one of the most amazing experiences of my life.

The week came to an end, and we pulled the boat out of the ocean, put it back on our trailer and took it home. I'm not really sure how long it took for the slip to become available; however, I think it was maybe about six months. This was just fine. We had time to sand and paint the boat, give it a lovely deep blue hull color, and go through the cockpit and cabin cleaning and painting anything we could. The size on the inside reminded me of an old VW Bus, just a couple of small beds, some storage, and some room to lounge about.

This was the dream. I would get home from work, and we could walk down to the harbor and be out on the bay in no time at all. The kids' friends would join us, we would have meals on the boat, and we were all learning how to sail.

Sometime, about a year after we had the boat in the water, Susie was helping me move our heavy sleigh bed around in our bedroom. She lifted and felt something not quite right in her back. After a series of doctor visits Susie underwent disk replacement surgery for her back. Susie has endured more than 15 years of multiple surgeries and excruciating back, hip, and sciatic pain that all started with that initial injury. By all means, this is Susie's story to tell; however, my story would not be complete without sharing its origin.

Unfortunately, this injury quickly halted Susie's ability to participate and enjoy being present on our sailboat. The constant motion of the boat, as well as the need to quickly move back and forth were just way too painful given the nature of Susie's injury.

Over the next four years Kendyl and I made a regular date of sailing every Thursday night. Quite often a group of her friends from high school, or my friends from work, would join us; however, more often than not it was just me and Kendyl. We would take the boat out of the harbor, raise the sail, and head out around the wharf and out to mile buoy, then sail down south a way past Black's Beach and back into the harbor. We became very adept at handling the sails, as well as dropping the mast to go under the bridge and back up into the upper harbor. After scrubbing the boat and tucking her in with all her sail covers, we would head over to Michoacán Taqueria and grab a couple veggie burritos and horchatas for a post sail dinner.

Cooper enjoyed our boat; however, it didn't always involve taking it out of the harbor. We had some really fun nights camping on the boat over the years. Cooper and I would take our dogs, Mona, and Anna, as well as our dinner and breakfast and set up camp in the boat for the night. I can remember each of us laying in our sleeping bags with our dogs tucked in, listening to the shrouds clang against the mast creating a meditative sound all through the night.

The sailing was lovely; however, for me, mostly, it was the human connection with my wife and children. Reminiscing on it feels like the proverbial ship-in-a-bottle. Time stood still while on the boat. Worries, stress, future, past; it all just faded away with the slowly rolling waves just off the Santa Cruz coast.

Tahoe

As I was discussing earlier, when stars align for both Susie and I on an idea, little can be done to stop it from happening. Such was the case during our family Thanksgiving trip to Tahoe the fall of 2005. One of my friends from work had set us up at the Tahoe Seasons for a Thanksgiving vacation. This whole concept was new to us, we had always had Thanksgiving with large family gatherings. The Tahoe Seasons was at the base of Heavenly Valley and snow was in the forecast so we thought we would give it a go and see how it went.

The kids were now 6th and 8th grade and we hadn't been to the snow since we left Mt. Shasta over 10 years earlier. The trip carried with it some amazing fun experiences, as well as interesting family growth dynamics. First of all, our two middle schoolers were sharing the living room to sleep in and in between the living room and our bedroom was a hot tub with shudders. Interesting condo arrangement reminiscent of a 70's honeymoon suite. We, of course, made the best of it and had a blast using the room-adjoining indoor hot tub!

Not very often in recent history has Heavenly Valley had enough snow to be open from top to bottom during Thanksgiving. This year was an exception. Plenty of snow had fallen early on and I had the opportunity to rent some skis and get back on the snow for the first time in over a decade. This stirred something in me. My legs had distant memories of what it felt like to glide and turn on the snow. The chill on my face as well as the amazing views of the mountains and the lake. Oh my God, the lake. Such an incredibly beautiful view, surrounded by snow capped mountains, simply mesmerizing.

While I was up on the mountain, we had the opportunity to get the kids introduced to the mountain through an all-day snowboard lesson. Based upon their reaction when we went to pick them up after their day on the mountain, they both had a fantastic time. The pursuit of snow-boarding opportunities has become a lifelong passion for Kendyl, taking every opportunity available to strap on the board and head for powder. Cooper decided snowboarding wasn't his thing and a couple years later participated in a weeklong skiing course. Although skiing has not been Cooper's lifelong passion, his innate athletic ability shows through when I see him sliding and turning down the hill on his skis.

The most unfamiliar moment of this trip came at Thanksgiving dinner. We all went out to a casino, in search of a restaurant that would serve us the traditional dinner. We ended up in a not-so-fancy diner style restaurant in Harvey's Casino. The food was not bad, but we could tell the kids really missed having everyone around like we would back in Santa Cruz. The cousins, aunts, uncles, and other assorted friends were all missing. Susie and I did the best we could, with memories of gratitude and happy family conversation; however, Thanksgiving, in our family, definitely has a meaning of home, family and leftovers.

We woke Saturday morning to six inches of fresh snow on the roads. Absolutely serene and other-worldly. Susie and I got up early, left Cooper and Kendyl tucked into their couches and cartoons, and we headed down to Stateline to take a look at the new Heavenly Valley gondola that had just been built to transport skiers from the downtown condos directly up to the top of the mountain.

For over a year or so Susie and I had been ruminating about the idea of having some sort of vacation home. Susie had grown up with a vacation cabin in Tahoe, as I had talked about earlier; however, she made it clear she did not want to spend her vacations painting walls and cleaning gutters. For me, I just wanted to have some place I could go where it was just a short walk to a ski lift.

As we drove down to Stateline, it was definitely not our intention to be looking for some sort of family vacation property. The snow was gently falling, all of South Lake Tahoe was blanketed with this beautiful layer of fluffy powder. We could see the new gondola spinning around this amazing looking lodge type building in the middle of a newly developed Heavenly Village. We were speechless. This was not like any Tahoe we remembered or had grown up with.

After walking through the snowy dream for 15 minutes or so, we found ourselves touring the Grand Residence Club at the heart of the Heavenly Village. We walked into the 3rd floor apartment and felt like we were home. Standing in the living room, looking out over the courtyard swimming pool with the twinkling lights and snow falling, Susie and I were both all in. Within 60 minutes Susie and I were the proud owners of our new vacation condo, for one week each month December through April.

To say we (or at least me) didn't have any buyer's remorse would be a lie. Of course, I wondered if we had done the right thing. Susie, in her great wisdom, just kept reassuring me that we had done the right thing. For the first six or seven years, we used all our weeks every year. This had definitely become our second home. We would all get season passes, family ski days, and lots of friends.

When I take time to look back at my photo file of over 30,000 photos, I am amazed that nearly one-quarter of all my photos are of Tahoe trips. Tahoe had become a significant center for our family life, and still is today.

When I was a kid, our vacations were camping in Yosemite. For our kids, the Grand Residence Club Marriott was their camping place. We drive up to the valet, they welcome us back, take our luggage to our condo and park our car for us. When I say, Tahoe was their camping, I'm referring to the time and space. This location became second nature to our kids. They

148

were comfortable and safe running around and exploring Heavenly Village, they brought many different friends with them over the years, we had countless hours playing in the pool and sledding, and our move and game time back in the condo created memories that will last forever.

As the kids grew older and started their own lives, it became more difficult for them to get time away from their life to join us for five weeks each year. Susie and I, with our newfound knowledge of point trading, began trading for one of the larger condos so we could have a group of friends join us for a week each winter. It's amazing how well you can get to know your friends when you spend an entire week with them in a condo in the mountains. Both Susie and I have grown to look forward to these vacations and are looking forward to covid passing so we can once again safely gather a group of three or four other couples to join us for a week of entertaining in Tahoe.

For nearly 20 years Susie and I have had countless weeks where it is just Susie and I in our condo for the week. Absolutely wonderful get-away-date time. I'll usually get up and be on the mountain at first open, get in three hours of skiing and be back by lunch. We then proceed to spend the rest of the day hanging out with each other. Cross country skiing, walking, shopping, adventuring around Tahoe exploring; we never seem to tire of each other's company. We always love to make wonderful dinners and then hang out to watch a new series or movie. As fun as it is, by the sixth day we are ready to come back to our home in Santa Cruz.

Dropping into Killebrew Canyon, snow up to my armpits, so steep I'm floating for 20 feet before I regain pressure under foot just long enough to turn and drop again. First tracks on Little Dipper, two feet of fresh powder sweeping over the bumps creating the smoothest bump run I'll ever experience. Screaming past the trees on a hard pack bobsled run through the Tamarack trees, knowing that I need to be looking three turns ahead to assure branches and trees are avoided. Standing at the top of the Fire Break, looking three thousand feet down toward South Lake, preparing to launch into a giant slalom through backcountry Tahoe crust, remembering to drive my shins forward, stay on my edges and float through each turn. Heavenly Valley has some of the most amazing skiing on the planet and I look forward to many more years of fun and adventure with family and friends.

22

Practicing Pharmacist

My first job in a pharmacy I learned there was a secret and foreign language pharmacists use to talk about medications. It was in 1982 in San Diego and I was a second-year freshman at San Diego State University. As a clerk at Alvarado Medical Arts Pharmacy, the pharmacist had a genuine authenticity about him. He was a real person, he cared for his patients, and he had this huge and complicated phone bank that was specifically for all of the doctors in the medical clinic to get ahold of him. Lights would flash and he would pick up one of the lines, knowing exactly who he would be conversing with. He then went on talking this completely unknown medical language, as if it were some sort of secret society. I wanted it and was willing to do what it took to get it. I quickly learned how to type prescriptions, stock pharmacy shelves, run accounts receivable and manage the front end of a small clinic pharmacy. This was fantastic. I enjoyed the interactions with customers, the comradery with my fellow employees and learning all I could about this unknown world of pharmacy.

As a first year pharmacy student, my next pharmacy job was working in an independent pharmacy in downtown Stockton. Unfortunately, the owner didn't want the pharmacy students doing any of the pharmacy work, mainly I was out front, stocking the shelves with stuffed animals and other gifts. This position didn't last long, maybe two months, when a position opened up at Fry's grocery store pharmacy. I quickly applied and was accepted as my first pharmacist intern position, smock and all. This position included typing, filling, counseling, and all sorts of real-life pharmacy activity. I was able to stay at this position for nearly 18 months until I was sent out on clinical rotations.

At University of the Pacific, clinical rotations involve participating in six different areas of pharmacy practice for six weeks each. Fortunately, I had the amazing opportunity of traveling to Hawaii and working in our program set up in the Tripler Army Medical Center on Oahu. There were eight of us pharmacy students, and we would meet each morning in the basement of this tremendously huge hospital in a tiny little office before we went off to our assignments for the day. Throughout the course of the year, we were exposed to all types of clinical, retail and administrative pharmacy practice.

During this time in Hawaii, one of my rotations took place in the Cardiac Care Unit. One of our duties as pharmacy students was to respond to the general area of the bedside whenever a code-blue was called. As a student, our main goal was to just observe and stay out of the way. The resident physicians and intern doctors were not looking at the pharmacy students for advice on what to do next. They had their protocol; however, it was important for us to see and experience how these events transpired. In one particular case, this lady in her late 90's was brought back to life after a few minutes of resuscitation. Next, the team decided to place a catheter down into her heart so they could better measure her heart function. As a teaching hospital, I'm not really certain if they were doing this to help ensure an improved quality of life for their patient, or, teaching an aspiring medical intern how to place this type of catheter. My point in talking about this is that she was looking at me and was in pain. I stepped forward, receiving approval from the resident physician, and reached out my hand. I held her hand while they poked and needled her for about 30 minutes. Her name was Mrs. Mooney and she was all alone on the island of Hawaii. Her husband was a retired navy man who had passed away some years earlier and she had no children or other family on the island. I could tell we connected, I learned a little bit about being present for patients, and she had someone's hand to hold for the last 30 minutes of her life. She coded again toward the end of her procedure and passed.

After graduation I moved back home to Ben Lomond, where I was able to begin an intern position with Boulder Creek and Felton pharmacies. The owner was extremely helpful in teaching me how an independent pharmacy operated. His knowledge of the community and ability to provide a needed service helped him build an incredibly successful business. The owner was in the local volunteer fire department. One of the days he received a call and left me in charge of the pharmacy. Maybe not the best idea because I was still an intern; however, this is how it worked in 1987 in rural Boulder Creek. He came back about two hours later, opened the back door behind the pharmacy to the bathroom and stepped into six inches of water. He turned, looked at me and said, "You didn't flush the toilet, did you?" This was an excellent job I had for about six weeks while I was studying for the state board of pharmacy exam.

Upon taking the California State pharmacy exam, I packed up and moved to Boston, where I took and passed the Massachusetts State pharmacy exam as well. My first real life pharmacy position was at Osco Pharmacy in Everett, MA. My supervisor, who at the time was 27 years old, was a seasoned and wise old pharmacist. After six months of 12-hour retail pharmacy shifts I was questioning why I ever went into pharmacy as a profession. This was absolutely not what I had envisioned for my life of pharmacy practice. Inorder to continue my life as a pharmacist, I needed a change.

Securing a hospital pharmacy position at Community Hospital of Santa Cruz, I packed up and left Boston. Hospital pharmacy practice was completely different from the world of chain-store retail pharmacy. I absolutely loved the atmosphere, work, and responsibility. Quickly I became confident in running the hospital pharmacy while also providing drug information to the patients, nursing staff and physicians in the hospital. As well, during this time, I worked a couple three hour morning shifts each week at Mission Street Pharmacy. The owner had varicose veins terribly bad and spent most of his time in the back of the pharmacy with his legs elevated on a stool. I would come in the morning and help him get out as much work as I could. Interestingly, he still worked with an old manual typewriter. I would pack my small Epson portable electric typewriter and bring it with me anytime I went in to do a shift.

Within 18 months I had moved again, now practicing at Mt. Shasta Community Hospital as a staff pharmacist, leading into a director of pharmacy position, all of which lasted six years. These were the years when I really learned how a hospital pharmacy worked. I was able to participate in clinical as well as regulatory activities with an ever-increasing responsibility.

As a young hospital pharmacist in Mt. Shasta I was eager to begin implementing some of the tools I had learned just a couple years back in my pharmacy rotations. At the time, drug usage review (called DUR) was the latest buzz phrase in hospital pharmacy. The process involves choosing one medication, based upon selected criteria, and then monitoring its usage in the hospital for three or four months.

Our director in the pharmacy had heard of this process; however, had yet to implement any studies thus far. He tasked me with coming up with a proposal, presenting it at committee, and then implementing the study. He may have not had any experience with this particular process; however, he was a master with his physician and nursing communication.

The outcome of over four years' worth of DUR studies was tremendously positive; however, it was the communication skills I learned along the way that created the greatest experience. The process involved direct interface with nursing and medical staff with each review. The process was designed to be educational, with positive patient outcomes always as the leading indicator. In addition, the goal of each review is to help direct prescribing habits toward the most cost-effective manner of utilizing any specific medication.

Importantly, before any short consultation with a physician, define for yourself what you would like the outcome to be. Have your desired plan, as well as an alternative plan ready to go. The key to a successful clinical intervention is to present the situation, clinically and concisely, followed directly with the outcome you would like to see happen. Over the years I

154

have found that 10-15 minutes of quality research, prior to any two minute interface with a doctor, will most always lead to a reasonable and mutually acceptable clinical plan.

Shortly after I began as a pharmacist at Mercy Mt. Shasta I heard over the intercom, code-blue ER. My supervisor, Ron, looked at me and said, let's go Steve. My heart was pounding out of my throat with adrenalin; however, Ron was as casual as ever. We walked into a rapidly boiling emergency room with a team of people moving around the gurney. The crash cart had already been pulled into the room and a nurse was beginning to take the medication tray out of the cart when Ron stepped up and said, clearly and confidently, "I'll take that". I quickly realized, our job is to manage the medications. The physician runs the code, everyone else has their tasks, and the pharmacist manages the medications, period. I don't recall the outcome of that particular code; however, over the next six years at Mercy Mt. Shasta I attended at least 50 code-blue events. My job was to keep the medications ready, anticipate which medication was going to be used next and have it ready, keep track of the time between doses of specific medications, and be ready with my calculator for any quick dosing recommendations. As time passed, I became much more comfortable with my skill set and was able to enter the event with the calm demeanor my supervisor had once shown me.

Upon returning to Santa Cruz, I began working at Tom's Medical Clinic Pharmacy at the Santa Cruz Medical Clinic. This was to be a temporary position until the Sutter Maternity and Surgery Center opened for business. I was signed on to be the Director of Pharmacy for the new hospital. While at Tom's pharmacy, I rotated between the West Side pharmacy and the Main store. Life was a little chaotic at this time so I cannot give a real good beat on the work environment; however, I can say that Tom senior, and later ,his son, Tommy, run an incredibly vital business for the medical clinic. Their service to patients is second to none. As we talked about earlier, just prior to the hospital opening for business, I turned myself in to my supervisor for stealing and using drugs, asked for help, and entered rehabilitation.

Eighteen months later I began working at Dominican Hospital. Looking back on it, all of the work I did prior to rehab was preparing me for my work at Dominican. I was hired on as a per diem pharmacist, picking up as many shifts as I could in the hospital pharmacy. After about six months of work, a full-time position opened up in the out-patient store. I applied for the position and worked there for the next 25 years.

Throughout my practice I spent over 32 years working for Dignity Health, previously known as Catholic Healthcare West, and most recently known as Common Spirit Health. The first seven years were in the inpatient hospital pharmacy, and the last 25 had been in the outpatient clinic pharmacy located on the Dominican Hospital campus.

How incredibly fortunate I was to have a position in the pharmacy profession where I could work from 9-5:30, five days per week, and be present for my family while the kids were growing up. I started in this particular position when our children were in preschool and kindergarten, which allowed me to always have my evenings and weekends free for school and family events.

As a clinic pharmacist for a community hospital, I had the opportunity to be part of the hospital team, working with the doctors, nurses and patient care coordinators. Throughout the day I would coordinate with the hospital team to assure patients received their medications and appropriate education before they were discharged.

As well, being a small community pharmacy, we had the opportunity to develop relationships with our customers, know them by name, and be available for them to call with questions anytime during the day. Through this community pharmacy practice, I have come to feel very passionate about educating patients and caregivers about their treatments.

This passion for patient education led me to develop an online consumer medication information platform called AudibleRx. For more than 10 years, in the early morning hours before work, I developed this platform. Initially by myself; however, as time passed I took on a partner and some web and marketing help. With nearly 300 education sessions built in two languages, recorded and available for free on our website, we were meeting an educational need for those challenged with literacy or visual impairment. After 12 years of development, we donated the entire platform to a non-profit organization who works with hundreds of hospitals across the country.

Throughout my years at Dominican I was given the opportunity to develop and implement many clinical programs and continue to enhance my learning through educational opportunities. One thing we all know for certain, nothing ever stays the same. Like many industries, the outpatient pharmacy business model has come up against some steep barriers to successful operation over the past decade.

Unfortunately, outpatient pharmacy practice has traditionally been considered a product-service industry, as opposed to a clinical-service. Product-service business models base their success on their ability to provide products at a competitive price. Clinical-service models look specifically at the outcome of their patient population to determine how successful they are at providing their service. Of course, this is an incredibly simplistic way of looking at an overly complex topic; however, you get the idea.

Every day our store would fill a certain number of prescriptions. This number becomes the metric which our productivity is based on. Of course, after some time, we are faced with how to continue to meet that same productivity number with fewer resources. Over the last few years at my outpatient pharmacy position, this process continued to cycle. We became incredibly efficient at filling prescriptions; however, our clinical consulting time with patients became diminished as our need to meet our company metrics increased.

For me, personally, I found myself regularly thinking about what life would feel like if I did not need to come into the store every day and fill prescriptions. It had been an excellent job for quite some time; however, I felt my happiness slowly draining from my soul.

With property values doing so well in Santa Cruz, Susie and I had been discussing, for a couple of years, the idea of selling and retiring somewhere outside of California. We produced a list of different locations and settled on a cute little town in Colorado, close to where some good friends live. Just to make the process complete, I went through the process of preparing for and taking the pharmacy exam for Colorado in order to become a licensed pharmacist in that state.

Susie could feel I was becoming increasingly unsatisfied with my work life. The thing is, we were not quite ready to make the move. Our son was living in our cabin in our backyard and was planning on getting married within a year, and we wanted to provide time and space to be present for this exciting event. After the wedding, our son and his newlywed bride moved into our cabin with plans on staying for at least two years, and the thought of sharing our property with them far outweighed our need to pack up and move somewhere else.

As often happens, when you are present for those around you, unexpected opportunities emerge. I received an email describing a part time pharmacist position becoming available at the other hospital in Santa Cruz, Sutter Maternity and Surgery Center. I was familiar with the institution, I had practiced as a part-time on-call pharmacist here for over 13 years earlier in my career; however, this was different.

The position was listed as part-time, only five days every two weeks; however, it came with full health benefits. Susie and I discussed it, and we came to the conclusion there's no way we'd be able to survive regular life in Santa Cruz and all that it costs working only half time. Then, shortly after our discussion, sitting at my desk late one night, an epiphany landed in my lap.

Following a deep dive into our retirement account, we concluded that, at 58 years old, I was eligible to officially retire from Dominican Hospital. After some long discussions with Susie and meaningful consultations with our retirement representative, we concluded the retirement package from Dominican, in addition to part time work, would allow us to sustainably maintain our Santa Cruz home while beginning the next phase of our life.

Now, the only barrier was to apply and be accepted for the position. It had been over 25 years since I had interviewed for a job, so I was a bit nervous. Fortunately, the interview went beautifully and within a few weeks I was giving my notice at Dominican and preparing to begin a position as a part time inpatient pharmacist at Sutter hospital.

Interestingly, during my interview, I found I treated it similar to how I had treated my interview at Dominican over 25 years earlier. I led with my story of sobriety. Perhaps I could have left it unsaid, especially because I have now been sober for more than 27 years; however, in my humble opinion, which would have left me feeling just a little bit less than honest. Having the discussion, up front and center, set the stage for a truly genuine discussion about my goals, as well as an understanding of the specific set of tools I bring with me into the practice of pharmacy.

As part of the interview, we discussed the bedside education and medication reconciliation process. Excitedly, this was a program the hospital was hoping to implement, and the director of pharmacy was now asking me if I would be interested in participating in developing the process. As I was discussing earlier, through my time at Dominican, twice I had implemented this type of program, and both times the program had been canceled after six months due to lack of funding. Sutter was now interested in beginning this type of program and assured me it will become part of the daily function, not just a 6-month trial program awaiting official funding. It has been over 12 months since I began my position here at Sutter hospital and yes, we now have a fully functional, staffed, and operational bedside education program in place.

The skill sets necessary for hospital pharmacy are, for the most part, significantly different from those of retail pharmacy. If it weren't for my initial seven years of hospital pharmacy practice at the beginning of my career, I don't believe the transition to where I am today would have been so smooth.

As you may recall from the chapter on cooking, Cooper had begun working at Sutter hospital as a cook and has been here for just over 10 years now. Cooper has developed relationships with just about everyone in the hospital, from the surgeons and anesthesiologists, the nursing staff, administrators, and all of the facilities management workers. As happens, when I am having conversations with other employees at the hospital, somewhere during the conversation they realize I am Cooper's dad. Without hesitation, absolutely everyone I come in contact with has nothing but wonderful things to say about Cooper.

As an "exit plan", this part time job gets as close as we can imagine to the perfect scenario. For quite some time, I had imagined that I would most likely retire somewhere around 65 years old. At that time, we had budgeted into our life that I would continue to work, maybe two days per week, at some pharmacy in order to stay current, pay for fun, and keep active in the pharmacy world.

With the advantage of full health benefits, beginning this process at 58 years old felt incredibly attractive and fortunate. After working here for nearly two years, the pace and workload lend itself to that balanced sense of sustainability which leads me to think I'll be here for quite some time.

***

Similar to just about any college degree an individual can get, pharmacy school and internships do not train an individual to practice pharmacy, they merely provide you with the tools necessary to obtain your first job as a pharmacist. Like absolutely everything, the practice of pharmacy is constantly evolving in many exciting directions.

The fall of 1978 was the highlight of my football career. I was in my sophomore year of high school, playing for the Junior Varsity team. As a defensive back, I had somehow come into my own that year with five interceptions, one of which I ran back for a touchdown. I can remember how exciting it felt to be confident in my actions, ability, and performance.

The following year I moved up to Varsity and it just wasn't the same. After a couple weeks of practice and the jamboree, I was relegated to second string receiver and special teams. For years I have credited my junior and senior year poor football statistics to my size. I was not big, at about 5' 8" and 150 pounds I was about the same size as my buddy, the field goal kicker.

As an individual beginning my third trimester of life, I now realize it had absolutely nothing to do with my size. Today, I am a firm believer that my football performance during my last two years of high school had everything to do with my lack of practice. All summer long prior to the 1979 season I did absolutely nothing to prepare myself for the upcoming year. One of my closest friends was the quarterback. I could have easily gone out and practiced running plays and drills with him. We could have built a trust so that when he threw the ball to me, he would trust that I would be there to catch it.

More than practicing drills, I could have done the leg work on my own. I could have practiced my sprints to assure I would have the speed necessary to get down the field, while also working on my endurance to assure I would be in top physical condition the entire game. It was not my size that limited my game, it was my lack of passion.

After nearly 4 decades of pharmacy practice, I feel it has just been over the past 15 years that I am beginning to reach my potential. Don't get me wrong, I have worked very hard over the years, it's just that I had never really found my passion in the game.

In my opinion, the pharmacy world has an abundance of extremely qualified pharmacists. We are excellent technical and tactical performers with incredible attention to detail. Clinically, we are second to none, prescribe appropriate follow up in all scenarios and are comfortable with medication education discussions with medical and nursing staff. We are perfectly adept at patient counseling, understand that different patients require different levels of education and are fluid and dynamic enough to overcome individual patient barriers and provide the information necessary to complete a medication counseling session at the pharmacy counter.

Over the years, pharmacists have moved from behind the counter, out to where the patient is, providing needed medication counseling. We have moved from the basement of hospitals, up to the patient floors, providing clinical education for medical and nursing staff and recommendations on patient care. Pharmacists now provide medication therapy management and vaccination services during house calls. In some facilities pharmacists are regularly involved in patient rounds and visit patients at their bedside prior to discharge. Pharmacists are achieving provider status. These are but a few of the avenues that pharmacy has expanded over the past few decades.

Absolutely none of this advancement would have happened if it weren't for pharmacists promoting and advocating for the profession of pharmacy. These are pharmacists who have found a passion in their work and are not afraid to talk about it. They bring their passion home with them and live with it 24 hours a day. For these individuals, pharmacy is not just a job; it is a calling, to move the profession forward while providing a needed service.

23

Stay Present

As a human on planet earth, I have come to believe in acceptance; right now, this exact moment, everything is exactly as it is meant to be. I may not like or agree with it; however, my simple disagreement will not change this specific moment. I have also come to believe in choice and action as tools I may implement if I ever find a moment I do not like or agree with. I accept and resolve to take responsibility for my own actions and the outcome of these actions are a direct reflection of my integrity.

For many years I have been working in pharmacies as a clean and sober pharmacist. My first day, walking into a pharmacy clean and sober, I began a ritual that I maintain each and every day. I always park far from the entrance to my workplace so that I may have a little bit of a walk to reach the door. As I am walking into the pharmacy, I have three prayers I say, slowly, to myself.

- 3rd Step Prayer
  - o God, I offer myself to Thee, to build with me and to do with me as thou wilt. Relieve me of the bondage of self, that I may better do Thy will. Take away my difficulties, that victory over them may bear witness to those I would help of Thy power, Thy love, and Thy way of life, may I do Thy will always.
- 7th Step Prayer
  - o My Creator, I am now willing that you should have all of me, good and bad. I pray that you now remove from me

every single defect of character which stands in the way of my usefulness to you and my fellows. Grant me strength, as I go out from here, to do your bidding.

- Serenity Prayer
    - o God, grant me the serenity to accept the things I cannot change, the courage to change the things I can, and the wisdom to know the difference.

I then add in my own short reminder: God, please help me do what I'm supposed to do and say what I'm supposed to say, I know I'm going to forget and need your help, amen.

Over the past 25 years, maybe I have missed a day, but I really don't think so. There have been times when I remember just before walking in the door and I stop outside for 30 seconds to run through the prayers. Over the years I have been involved in quite a few challenging situations. Never have I had a circumstance I wasn't able to manage in some sort of appropriate way.

Always Be Present.

24

These Days

Like many tasks or skills, I believe anyone can do just about anything if they practice, daily. In my humble opinion, this goes for writing as well. I'm not saying an individual will become an accomplished, published or even a good writer; however, with daily practice, they will definitely become a writer.

Over the course of writing this chronicle I have learned my memories are much more abundant than I give myself credit for. When sitting at a keyboard, thinking about a time and space in my life many years ago, I can see the thoughts go deeper and deeper as I wiggle my way into a memory. Then, I will get up and go sit with Susie, or one of my children if they happen to be around and share the memory with them. Quite often, just me discussing it with them takes the memory deeper and unleashes more information on the particular topic.

This idea of sharing my take on a distant memory, and then getting input on the memory from my family who were also present during the making of this particular memory, is an amazing way to create loving and even sometimes healing connections with each other. Such memories bring up these unsolicited emotions, which at times, may either be welcome, or, sometimes difficult to deal with. Maybe the difficult ones require a bit more time, to follow the memory through to the point where the emotion was resolved; or perhaps now is the time we get to go through it and resolve it.

***

These days Susie and I have developed an amazing Sunday morning ritual; we float on our couch. I'm not exactly sure how we came up with the term, float; however, it works for us. We sit, with our backs to the side of the couch and our feet up, looking at each other. Quite often our legs are entwined with each other in order for us both to fit comfortably this way on the couch.

When either one of us uses the "float" expression, we know exactly what the other means. This is our space for open communication. We'll use it for loving expressions, happy concerns, financial or family issues; it really doesn't matter, if one of us would like to discuss it, this is the place where we can work it out.

Come to find out, after all these years, Susie and I are really great friends. We both absolutely love creating a romantic dinner at home, maybe some ballroom dancing in the living room and a great movie. Years ago, pre-sobriety, when Susie and I were in couples therapy, the counselor told us we had the potential to have an amazing relationship. Today, I have the relationship I always dreamed about but never knew existed. Together, we enhance each other's strongest attributes and help each other out with the rest. It isn't as if we plan this; it's just that as time passes, our relationship gets stronger and more cohesive. Susie and I feel very fortunate to have each other.

Since our first date, more than four decades ago, we have been a fixture in each other's lives. There were a few years early on when I was away at college and we each had our own path; however, whether it was fate, coincidence, destiny, providence, or just plain love, our souls crossed paths once again. I am absolutely positive I would not be the man I am today if it were not for the loving kindness of my lovely bride. Some would think we are entering our senior years, well, that may actually be the case; however, we feel as if we are getting ready to start an exciting and new phase of our life.

166

Susie has taught me what it feels like to be desired. Not just physically, but emotionally and spiritually as well. Such an amazing feeling, understanding how another individual, whom you have known for well over 40 years, still desires to experience you more intimately. Of course, our mutual experience continues to encourage my growth and understanding of my passion for Susie. This is a constantly moving cycle, forever learning.

Over 30 years ago, before anyone knew how important it was, Susie was searching out organic food. At the time, I didn't understand the importance. Fortunately for me, that didn't slow down Susie's desire to feed us healthy meals prepared from organically sourced ingredients. Susie has a passion for learning. Her library of alternative healing, healthy cooking, and life balancing books is tremendous, and she will regularly think of something, step out of the room, and come back with a book to back up her thoughts.

My gratitude to Susie for bringing all of this into our lives is immense. School taught me how medicine may heal. Susie, over the years, helped me learn how our lifestyle, thoughts, feelings, emotions, surroundings, and nutrition may be more important at maintaining sustainable health than any western medicine may provide.

As I have described earlier, Susie was there for me and our family when we needed her most. She held the fabric of our family together, on her own, for quite a few years, while I was under the influence of drugs. Then, she trusted me to help create our family circle after I had learned how to live sober. What I didn't express is how she gave me the opportunity to be present for her when she needed me. Over the past 25 years Susie has experienced the heartbreak of losing family and the physical agony of pain.

Through the loss of grandparents and a loving sister, Susie has given me the opportunity to be present for her, allowing me to hold and comfort her in her most vulnerable moments. Additionally, she has undergone multiple spinal surgeries and has lived with ongoing physical pain for years. Throughout these years, most mornings, she wakes with a lovely smile on her face, a cheerful good morning, and a kiss for her husband. Despite the pain, she continues moving forward, creating gatherings of friends and family.

Anyone who has spent 60 minutes alone talking with Susie knows that she is one of the most empathetic and understanding individuals on this planet. Her ability to help whomever she is talking with feel completely relaxed and at home is a skill we should all aspire to. Susie has helped me learn how to listen. Not just hear what someone is saying, but quietly listen to the message they are sharing with me, and then repeat it back just to assure I understand them completely.

Over the years, and more so recently than in the past, we have begun reading in bed at night. Well, mostly it is about me reading and Susie listening. What an enormously enchanting way to connect. The thing is, after about 10 minutes of reading I can hear Susie with her tiny little sleepy breathing. Maybe I stop reading for just a moment to see if she is asleep or maybe still listening. Somehow, even though I am sure she is sound asleep, the moment I stop reading and prepare to set down the book, Susie's eyes pop open and ask if the chapter is over. "Well, no it's not over silly, you were sleeping", so I pick up and continue reading, with a comforting smile on my face and a warm heart.

This morning, after floating on the couch for a couple hours, we packed up and drove north of Santa Cruz up to Wilder Ranch. The sun was shining on this Halloween day, with just a little breeze in the air, and we could smell the ocean a half a mile away. Walking hand in hand on the trail, we could feel the ocean getting closer with every step; with each of us feeling the enormity of how superbly beautiful our hometown really is.

It is incredibly fulfilling, realizing that year after year, we are both able to understand, care for, and love each other more completely than the year before. Over the coming weeks, months, and years we will have many opportunities to be present for each other. With our deep trust and interconnectivity, I am positive all of our years will be filled with emotional, spiritual, and physical opportunities for us to be present for one another.

Made in the USA
Middletown, DE
10 December 2024

66540267R00099